Good Luck To Elaine Doran
at Bel...

C000090658

Published by
SSJT Publishers
Kent, UK

First Edition
November, 2006
All rights reserved

ISBN
0-9554511-0-8
978-0-9554511-0-2

Cover design © Roopina

Printed and bound in India by **Big Satisfaction**
bsatis@rediffmail.com

Foreword

The great thing about Dr Singh's weight loss programme is its simplicity. No calorie counting, no special diet foods, no expensive equipment.

In his book, inspired by his father's death from a heart attack, Dr Singh draws on his experiences as a GP and as a son. He deplores the way that our high-fat, high-sugar, processed diet has made obesity and coronary heart disease commonplace and says we are poisoning ourselves with bad food.

He also questions our custom of eating (or over-eating) three times a day, regardless of whether we are hungry.

Dr Singh regards conventional dieting - with its calorie counting, detoxing and 'slimming' potions - as a short-term fix. Long-term weight loss, he argues, means, simply, making healthy eating a habit. Simple as this may sound, it's not boring.

Susan Fenton
Features Editor, Progressive Housewares magazine.
BA Hons (Humanities); Certificate in Newspaper Journalism (National Council for the Training of Journalists); Diploma in Public Relations (Communications, Advertising and Marketing Foundation); member National Union of Journalists.

Editor

Susan Fenton is a freelance journalist with a personal interest in healthy eating and weight loss. She is features editor of Progressive Housewares, a business magazine which covers the areas of cooking and healthy eating.

She has been a writer on regional newspapers and international business magazines and has been a freelance sub-editor on national newspapers. She has also edited staff magazines for major corporations and has done book copy-editing.

Susan is a member of the National Union of Journalists and has professional qualifications in journalism, public relations, marketing communications and industrial editing.

She is also a member of the Ramblers' Association, which gives her a special interest in Dr Singh's views on walking as a route to health.

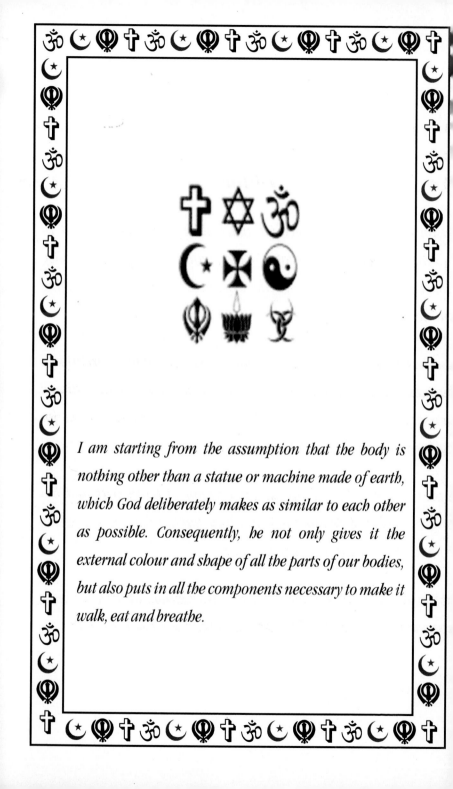

I am starting from the assumption that the body is nothing other than a statue or machine made of earth, which God deliberately makes as similar to each other as possible. Consequently, he not only gives it the external colour and shape of all the parts of our bodies, but also puts in all the components necessary to make it walk, eat and breathe.

From the author's desk

Writing this book has been a real pleasure for me. This book is written under Hippocratic Oath. If I had not written this book I would have been guilty of not letting people know the truth that I already knew. I was just seeking for a way to express my views. Since I was not practicing medicine I didn't have the opportunity to spread this knowledge with my patients. Whilst carrying on my studies and working, I did not have enough time to organise seminars.

This was the only way in which I could help people on what is the most controversial and ever-increasing health problem. We hear in the news every day about this deadly problem, but no one has the solution. I found this as a meagre problem, which I have tried to explain and unravel, through my first book "Healthy Heart". Earlier trials showed 65% success for the people who have understood the principle and theories mentioned in the book. If you have problems understanding some of the medical phrases in the book, you can come back to them later on. I promise you that it will make sense after all.

Health workers have the same prevalent rate of health illness as the general public; this book will undoubtedly be a helping hand to even themselves and their patients. Having said all this, please do not take the contents of my book as a prescription. Nevertheless, I would pledge you to treat it as an informative self-help book.

Special mentions to Sue Morgan, who chose the title, Susan Fenton di
the editing and the British Heart foundation for kindly allowing me

add one of their recent posters in this book.
I could not have accomplished this book without the help, motivatio
and support of my wife. She has been with me throughout the thick a
thins of this experience. This book is the secret to having her cook
meals everyday.

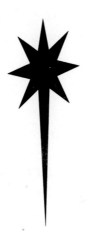

Dedicated to my father, I will miss him always.

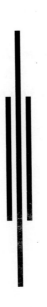

My Promise

I promise that in this book I will not advise any strenuous exercise regime, no unappetising-looking, cardboard-like diet, and no miraculous pills.
Your promise

All I need you to say is:

"I promise to stay healthy all my life"

Hold my hand and I will take you to the.……….................

STARS

Universe

Where we belong, where we have our home, our family and all the people we love.

From now on, if you write down your address as the universe and understand completely what I say, everything will become easy to understand. You will not be narrow minded to believe in race, caste, culture, religion, boundaries and borders. Once in a while, relax and you will think that is the absolute truth.

What has happened is that we are taught into it. We are motivated in such a way that we cannot think in our own way, we have to do what we are taught to do. We think the way that we are taught to think, and we believe what we are taught to believe. We are brainwashed to having three meals and believe that we cannot miss a meal. We are told that we have to have five portions of fruit a day. I would ask that you start believing in yourself and start thinking by yourself.

I know it is hard to break centuries of customs and traditions; still this is my desperate plea, to try to improve for your health.

What we have is centuries of belief in food. What we have forgotten is that the manufacturer of this sophisticated machine, the human body, has provided us with the brain that we think with.

We can smell and identify the edible food.

We can taste and tell whether we can eat that food or not.

If we can see and decide which food is edible, then why do we have to believe in someone telling us that food which was considered inedible can be eaten by certain processing methods?

Earth

Earth is one of the planets out of millions in the universe. This is the only planet where life is feasible.

The first dinosaurs lived on this earth about 230 million years ago. Dinosaurs ruled this earth. They were everywhere on this earth. Some of them were birds and they flew, some were huge and walked on earth, some of them were swimmers and they lived for millions of years. Some of them were vegetarians, some were meat eaters and they fought with each other. They looked after their families. They had every feature in their bodies with which to fight nature's disasters, so they had thick skin to protect them against bad weather, they had horns to break things, and they had teeth to chew.

About sixty millions years ago they vanished and no one knows quite what happened to them. I can only assume that if they had continued to exist, then there would have been very little vegetation left over for us to live on.

Fortunately, some of them managed to survive, for example:

Crocodile, hippopotamus and tortoise

Dinosaurs

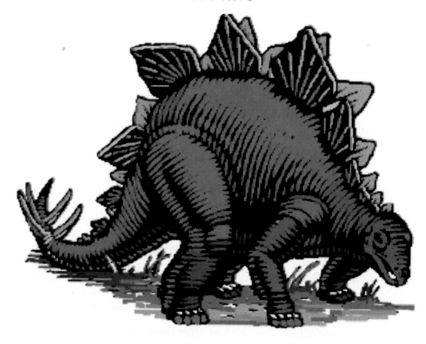

Crocodile

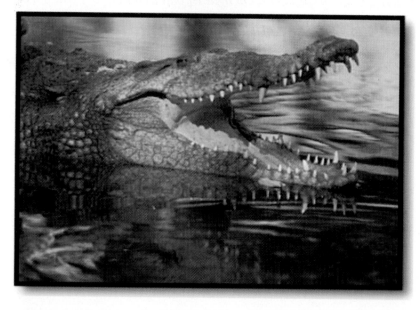

Tortoise

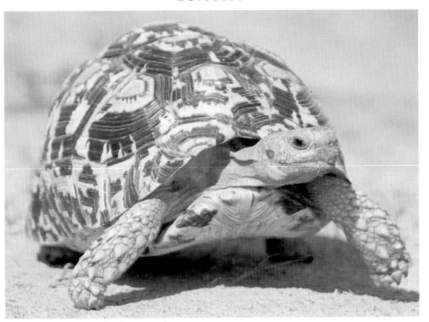

Hippopotamus

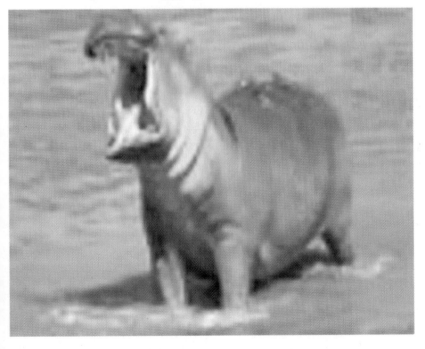

Theory of evolution

Are we the product of dinosaurs? I am afraid I have to disagree with that idea. Are we aliens on this earth? Just a thought! If that is the case then where did we, as human beings, originate?

According to the theory of evolution, we travelled a long journey from amoeba to human beings. Charles Darwin says we are the generation of the monkey, and we have adapted ourselves according to the environment and our needs.

Homosapien

We human beings belong to a sub-class of mammals. We are the class of vertebrate animals characterized by the presence of hair and the presence of mammary glands, which in females produce milk for the nourishment of the young. We have warm-blooded bodies, we have four appendages, a four-chambered heart and we have hairy skin. Our body structure is made up of three constituents: air (gas), earth (solid) and water (liquid).

Muscles, bones and other body organs are made of the same matter as other vegetation on this earth. Our bodies are estimated to be about 60 to 70% water. Water keeps the blood in a liquid state that provides the means for nutrients to travel to all our organs. Our muscles, lungs, and brain all contain a large amount of water.

Nenandra

This man has no worries in the world. He does not have to worry about going to work. He does not have to pay bills or a mortgage. His greatest worry is food. Does he have enough for now, for today, and when will he run out of the food? After millions of years, this concern is still on our conscious and it is in our nature as human beings that we think of food twenty times a day, even though food has been around us in abundance, since the beginning of time. The producer of this sophisticated machine has provided us with the full supply, only we do not distribute it evenly. The result of this is that some are suffering from starvation and others are suffering from overeating.

Our Neolithic ancestors were a very advanced race and by about 5,000 BC they had changed from their nomadic lifestyle of hunting and gathering. The influx of agriculturists from the East led to a more settled lifestyle, based on farming communities, as new skills were learned and passed on.

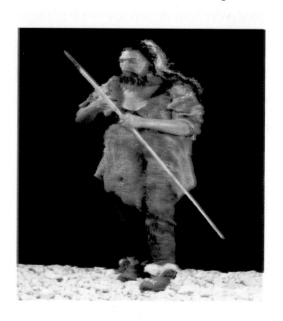

Breathing

The process of taking air in and out to the lungs through the nose is called The Respiratory System. The primary function of the respiratory system is to supply the blood with oxygen, in order for the blood to deliver oxygen to all parts of the body. The respiratory system does this through breathing. When we breathe, we inhale oxygen and exhale carbon dioxide. This exchange of gases is the respiratory system's means of getting oxygen to the blood. As long as this process is repeated we are alive.

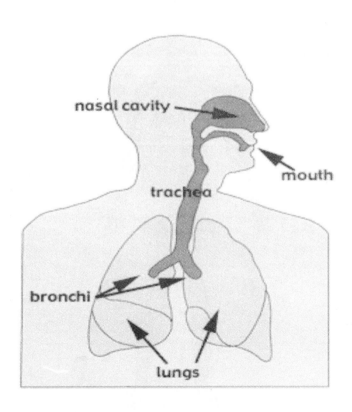

Blood circulation

On average, your body has about 5 litres of blood continually travelling through it by way of the Circulatory System. The heart, lungs and the blood vessels work together to form the circular part of the circulatory system. The pumping of the heart forces the blood on its journey through the body taking the oxygen and other nutrients to the functioning parts. The beating of the heart is a clear indicator that you are alive.

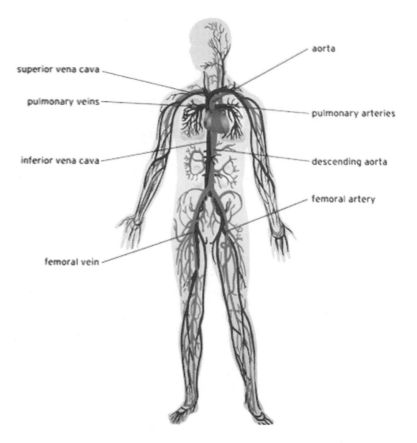

Digestive system

Everything we eat is grinded, crushed and mixed in our stomach.

Very simply, the digestive process is the means by which food is taken into our bodies. It is used to provide us with energy and nutrients like proteins, carbohydrates, vitamins, minerals and water. These are taken out and kept, as they are needed for growth, renewal and distributed in the body. Anything that is not used is kept in the end of the intestinal canal and taken out as defecation. This whole process takes about twenty-four hours.

All of this takes place in the 'gastro-intestinal tract'. The total length of the digestive tract is an amazing nine metres.

This process starts at the mouth where food enters the body and ends at the anus where waste leaves the body.

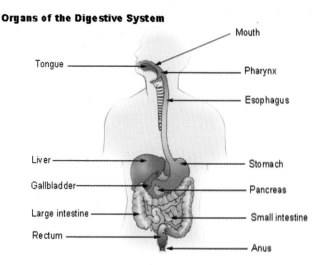

Organs of the Digestive System

Hunger

Hunger is applied literally to the feel, need or craving for food. The uneasy sensation of hunger is caused by a lack of food. It is a queasy sensation in our stomach that tells us we have run out of fuel and that we need some more. It has a reflex from our brain, which can be conditioned with taste, smell and look. Some feel starved and some feel sick. A rumbling sound in the stomach makes you think that something is wrong: in fact, it is a normal physiological phenomenon.

Thirst

Thirst is a physiological need to drink. The feeling of thirst is similar to a hunger sensation: a dry mouth, a feeling of need and craving. When we feel these sensations we cannot decide whether they are of hunger or thirst: most of the time they are of thirst rather than hunger.

Dehydration

Even before you start to feel thirsty, you are already partially dehydrated; drinking water regularly throughout the day will make sure you are taking in enough liquid.

People of all age groups can be affected by fluid and electrolyte imbalance. However, infants and children are the group that are most at risk.

Normal tea, coffee and coke contain caffeine and fruit juices act as a diuretic, increasing the flow of urine, causing further dehydration.

Starvation

Starvation affects many systems of the body. These include physiological symptoms such as anaemia, low sodium, potassium and other elements including bradycardia, immunological deficiencies and arrhythmias. Most changes are completely reversible as weight is regained. David Blain survived 40 days without food without any major deterioration to his health.

Men

Men preserve their extra stores of food in their bellies and around the central parts of the body.

Women preserve their food around the lower section of their body. This is usually around the hips and bottom as a fat under the skin.

When this process continues, this means that there is more intake than consumption, which leads to a situation called obesity.

Food preservation

There are many species of animals that mainly eat stolen food, for example rats, bacteria and flies. Others who earn their food have to keep it for further use, so nature has provided us with the instinct to preserve food.

This preserved food can be used when needed and can be transferred into energy.

Every species has its own method of preserving food.

When these stores are depleted, these same stores need to be restored first. That is why, when your body is starving for food, you feel even hungrier after a meal.

Animal kingdom
Animal instinct is better than humans.

Lion

A lion eats animal meat as a staple diet. He kills the animal only when he is hungry. When he has eaten, he is very lazy and sleeps all day.

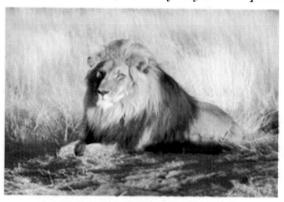

Elephant

An elephant eats vegetation and keeps on munching all day. He is very strong and a useful animal to human beings. He is an excellent method of transport and a good tool to work. Elephants are well known for their friendship to human beings.

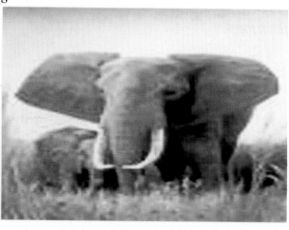

Vulture
A Vulture waits for the death of their victim.

Camel
Not knowing when he is going to find food next, a camel preserves his food in his hood/humps for days. He can survive without eating food for many days.

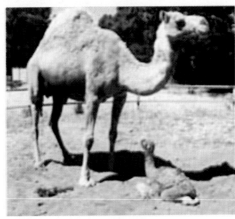

Squirrel

A squirrel only eats what is needed and rest of the food she stores in heaps. She moves and preserves her food in places where she thinks the food will be kept safe.

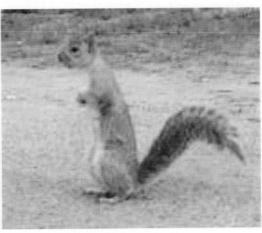

Why we over eat

I have explained why our anxiety about food availability is still in our thoughts and why we have to preserve some food for the future. One other factor is that food is very tasty and makes us greedy. When this happens too frequently we form the habit of consuming more than is needed. Over time the same quantity does not satisfy us, so we eat more. Our stomach is a bag of muscle, which can be stretched according to the need, but it is very hard to bring it back to its original size.

There are some other conditions, which lead us to overeat and result in obesity.

Depression

If you are feeling a bit stressful, anxious or depressive, then I know how you feel. It may feel as though nobody knows or even understands what you're going through. Often depression has no obvious cause. It can affect anyone at any time in their life, even during childhood, although it is more common in mid-life. At any one time, about one in 20 people suffer with clinical depression. Eating is sometimes the usual escape route. Usually with depression people do not move around a lot, which causes weight gain and which only adds to their worries. If you think you are depressed, the first thing to do is tell someone, especially your doctor, and get some help. There is no point in suffering in silence from this very painful condition.

In depression, people experience feelings of worthlessness and hopelessness. Physical illness or injury, headaches, digestive problems, pain, sadness, excessive crying and the loss of pleasure do not cause these ongoing physical problems. Sleeping too much or too little can also be a sign of depression, as well as low energy, restlessness, difficulty concentrating, irritability, thoughts of death and suicide.

Over eating can never be a solution for depression - rather, it will only add to your problems.

Boredom

Almost half of adults turn to food when they have feelings of boredom, loneliness and stress. We find eating an enjoyable pastime. In fact we are escaping from boredom when we indulge in eating.

Anxiety

Everybody feels anxious from time to time - it is a normal response to stressful situations.

Anxiety is a feeling of unease. Everybody experiences it when faced with a stressful situation, for example before an exam or an interview, or during a worrying time such as an illness. It is normal to feel anxious when facing something difficult or dangerous and mild anxiety can be a positive and useful experience.

However, for one in ten people in the UK, anxiety interferes with normal life. We switch to eating while we are waiting for something to happen, but this makes the situation worse.

Illness

There are some illnesses which can cause obesity. They are very rare and can easily be tested for. If you think that you have gained or lost weight recently and quickly, it is better that you get checked by your doctor and have a blood test.

Here are some examples.

Myxoedema

Myxoedema is a Thyroid-deficiency disease, which develops in adult life.

This is most common in middle-aged women. The symptoms include loss of energy, appetite, weight gain, and inability to keep warm, mental dullness, dry and puffy skin. Giving the thyroid hormone called thyroxin reverses the disease.

Cushing's syndrome

Cushing's syndrome is a group of bodily changes caused by an excess of steroid hormones. Taking medical steroid treatment over a long time usually causes this syndrome. This condition can also occur naturally. This is identified by weight gain around the chest and abdomen. The face becomes red and rounded, described as a moon face.

Hormonal imbalance

Pregnancy, Adrenal hyperplasia, Pituitary dysfunction and Polycystic Ovary syndrome, the usual symptoms are menstrual irregularities, weight gain, facial hairs, acne, hypertension and diabetes. Treatment is usually by a specialist doctor.

Medical treatment

Some of the medicine given by your doctor can lead to weight gain. Doctors usually warn you before giving them to you, such as steroids, antidepressants and contraceptives.

Obesity

Obesity is a condition in which the natural energy reserves of humans or other mammals stored as fat tissue is expanded far beyond usual levels to the point where it impairs health. Obesity in wild animals is relatively rare, but it is common in domestic animals like pigs and household pets that may be overfed and under exercised. In humans it is considered a major challenge to health.

Not all obese people eat more than the average person, but all obviously eat more than they need to.

Complications of obesity

Diabetes mellitus, Dyslipidaemia, Hypertension, Proinflammatory state, Gallstones, Pancreatitis, Fatty liver, Structural Obstructive sleep apnoea syndrome, Gastro-oesophageal reflux, increased skin infections, Thromboembolic disease, Pseudotumour Cerebri, Stress incontinence.

Cancers of the Endometrial, Breast, Ovary, Cervix, Prostate, Colon, Pancreas and Renal cell.

Degenerative Arthritis, Heart failure, Diabetes, Cirrhosis, Alzheimer's disease, Psychological, Depression, Anxiety,
The list is endless.

I do not mean to scare you but that is the truth.

Obesity is one of the biggest killers out there.

It kills more people than any war. It has the greatest effect on our cardio vascular system, which causes premature death.

Heart

The UK has the highest level of heart disease in the world and the incidence and prevalence of heart failure continues to rise.

Overall we estimate that there are just fewer than 1.5 million men living in the UK who have had CHD (either angina or heart attack) and about 1.1 million women, giving a total of around 2.6 million. CHD has a higher prevalence in Indian and Pakistani men in the U.K than in the other British population.

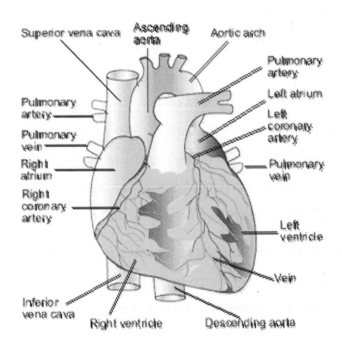

Heart disease

The overwhelming cause of coronary heart disease is atherosclerosis. This is a build-up of fatty materials within the walls of the arteries. This occurs when the inner lining of your artery walls become furred with a thick, porridge-like sludge (atheroma) made up of fatty deposits of cholesterol, cell waste and other substances. These form raised patches on the artery wall known as 'plaques' that narrow the arteries reducing the space through which blood can flow. At the same time, the blood becomes more prone to clotting.

The growing plaques may block the delivery of nutrients to the artery walls, causing them to lose their elasticity. This in turn may lead to high blood pressure, which also increases the risk of coronary heart disease.

A ruptured atheroma also may spill its fatty contents and trigger the formation of a blood clot (thrombus). The clot may further narrow or even occlude the artery, or it may detach and float downstream where it causes an occlusion (embolism), which stops blood supply to the heart and causes heart attack, most of the time it is fatal.

If it occludes the blood supply to the brain, it causes a stroke and if it causes the occlusion of vessels to the kidney, then this causes kidney failure. If it blocks the blood supply of limbs, then this results in the loss of limbs.

Arterioscleroses

What Causes Hardening Of The Arteries?

Blood vessels lose a certain amount of elasticity with aging. A build up of fatty deposits (plaque) occurs in the blood vessel lining.

Loss of vessel elasticity is termed arteriosclerosis, while fatty deposit build-up is termed atherosclerosis.

The process is thought to begin early in life.

Causative factors are: Cigarette Smoking, High Blood Pressure, Diabetes and Obesity.

The lipid is deposited in the in the artery. Fibrous plaques are raised firm pale areas in the artery, which on cross section reveal central lipid rich debris with surrounding fibrous tissue.

Fibrous Plaque

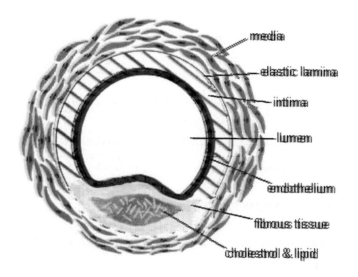

media

elastic lamina

intima

lumen

endothelium

fibrous tissue

cholestrol & lipid

Complicated plaques are raised fibrous plaques showing one or more of the following features.

Thrombosis.

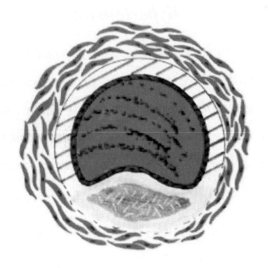

The formation, development or presence of a thrombus is an aggregation of blood factors, primarily platelets and fibrin with entrapment of cellular elements. It frequently causes vascular obstruction at the point of its formation.

Hypertension

High blood pressure is considered a major risk factor for a heart attack, heart failure and a stroke. About half of people having first-time heart attacks and two thirds of people having first-time strokes suffer from high blood pressure. Most cases of high blood pressure have no cure, but the overwhelming majority can be managed and controlled with diet and medication.

Vegetarians have lower blood pressures and healthier lipid levels in their blood.

Stroke

Stroke is the term used to describe the effects of an interruption of the blood supply to a localised area of the brain. If a part of the brain is deprived of blood, brain cells are damaged or die. This causes a number of different effects, depending on the part of the brain affected and the amount of damage to the brain tissue.

A majority of studies report that those who do regular to light to moderate activity have a lower incidence of stroke compared with those who are inactive, and some data suggests that vigorous activity confers no additional benefit.

Around 100,000 people in England and Wales have a stroke each year - one every five minutes. Nine out of 10 strokes affect people over the age of 55. 10,000 strokes a year occur in people under the age of 55. Some 300,000 people are living with disabilities caused by a stroke.

Case history

Age 61
Asian male
Height 5'11"
Weight 90 Kgs
Occupation retired engineer

Complained of discomfort in the chest in the middle of the night, and had a glass of water and went back to bed. After half an hour had a sudden pain in the chest, woke up, curled up and could not breathe. His son and daughter in law (both of them are doctors) sleeping in next bedroom ran to help him; they performed cardiac massage but could not revive him. Family doctor arrived within half an hour of the call and declared him dead. Cause of death was sudden cardiac arrest.

That's what I heard on the phone and I had to go to the funeral of my father. The reason I am telling you this story is that this is a typical story of a patient who dies of a heart attack, as only a few survive to tell the story themselves.

Anaemia

Anaemia is a condition in which the blood fails to supply the body's tissues with sufficient amounts of oxygen. The most common form of this condition is caused by iron deficiency.

The main cause of iron-deficiency anaemia is the loss of iron at a greater rate than normal as a result of abnormal persistent bleeding.

Another form of anaemia is due to deficiency of B12. It is caused when it cannot be absorbed from the intestinal tract mainly due to another hormone called intrinsic factor.

Eating disorder

Anorexia nervosa and bulimia is an eating disorder affecting mainly girls or women, although boys or men can also suffer from it. It usually starts in the teenage years. There is a strong, almost overwhelming, fear of putting on weight, with sufferers preoccupied with the shape or size of their bodies. Anorexia nervosa is self-induced weight loss caused by avoiding fattening foods and may involve taking excessive exercise, using laxatives or diuretics or self-induced vomiting.

Diabetes

Diabetes is a disease in which the body does not properly control the amount of sugar in the blood. As a result, the level of sugar in the blood is too high. This disease occurs when the body does not produce enough insulin or does not use it properly.

Diabetes can cause problems with the kidneys, legs and feet, eyes, heart, nerves, and blood flow.

If left untreated, these problems can lead to kidney failure, gangrene and amputation, blindness, or stroke.

Diabetes is on the increase, probably because people are living longer, getting fatter and leading increasingly inactive lifestyles.

Diabetes can't be cured, but it can be managed and kept under control. Anyone diagnosed with diabetes should seek treatment immediately to prevent associated illnesses.

Diabetes that occurs in middle age is called maturity onset diabetes. It is mainly controlled by diet control or some medication prescribed by your doctor. Weight control is a major issue in this type of diabetes.

Diabetes in younger age is usually treated by insulin injections. Insulin and diet go side-by-side depending on each other.

Change in either of them can cause serious side effects. Most people who have this diabetes are not over weight. Keeping a hold on their weight is the indication of control of their diabetes.

Autism (Autistic Spectrum Disorder, ASD)

Autistic children are more sedentary, so they are likely to put on weight and increase the problems for themselves, their parents and carers.

One advantage in autism is that autistic children are visual learners. They will learn the habits of people who they spend time with, whether these habits are eating food or exercise. It is easy to put an autistic child in a routine and it is hard to break their routine. It is very important that their routine is dealt with when they are younger.

Dieting

Following a diet of one kind or another is perhaps more common today than it has ever been. People commence diet plans for a wide range of reasons, including weight loss, increased energy, muscle growth, body repair, combating of illnesses and diseases, prevention of allergic reactions and avoidance of hyperactivity and depression. As you can see, the food you eat can have a profound influence on your physical and mental being.

There are a large number of diets available that can be tried and tested. Any type of dieting works. You can keep the weight off as long as you are on a diet; but as soon as you stop it is going to pile on again, resulting in a feeling of failure and sadness and thereby making the situation worse. And then you are going to choose another one and it is going to happen again.

Result:

Slippery slope.

Exercise

One of the main causes of obesity is lack of exercise.

If you are involved in any kind of sporting activity please carry on. If you are not doing any exercise please start today. Every kind of exercise is very good for health. It is as important as your food, water and oxygen.

You cannot control your weight by exercise alone.

All types of exercise involve using your muscles to generate movement. Regular exercise can increase muscle size, strength and endurance. But not all exercise produces the same effect.

Exercises like running or cycling make your muscles stronger and less likely to get tired. This sort of exercise doesn't only benefit your skeletal system. It also:

- *Enlarges your heart so it can pump blood around your body more quickly.*
- *Increases the capacity of your lungs so you can breathe in more oxygen with each breath.*
- *Improves your digestion.*
- *Makes your metabolism more efficient.*
- *Strengthens your skeletal system.*
- *Improves your coordination.*
- *Strengthens your immune system.*
- *Regular physical activity helps reduce the risk of developing complications of diabetes.*
- *Physically active people have a 33-50% lower risk of developing type 2 diabetes compared to inactive people.*

Here are some examples of exercises.

Indoor Exercise Items

Many products are available to buy, like indoor cycles, rowing and pumping machines, but most of them end up in the cellar or shed due to loss of interest in them. No doubt they are expensive items.

Bodybuilding and Weight lifting

Excessive muscle tone does not mean that someone is healthy or strong. A definition of health is completely different to that of the physique of a wrestler.

Health is not absence of disease also a state of mental, and social 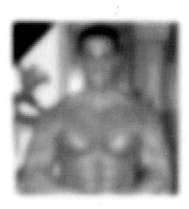 *merely the or injury, but physical, well-being.*

Vigorous activity additional benefit therapeutic value. *confers no to health and no*

Football

Football is a very good game. It teaches us discipline and teamwork, and also increases stamina and physical strength of the body. Almost every child has a dream of becoming the next David Beckham, but unfortunately disillusioned and their teenage years. clubs charge of money for their football is getting 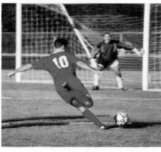 *millions get stop playing after These days, football enormous amount membership. But an increasingly bad reputation for football hooliganism.*

Swimming

A very good physical exercise, it increases strength, stamina and flexibility of the body. In my opinion every one should learn how to swim because of its beneficial effects on fitness, rather than it being a survival technique.

It takes about £1,000,000 to establish a community swimming pool and about £200,000 to build a pool in your back garden. You pay around £1,000 a year in membership fees to the sports club, plus the cost of daily visits. Many of us who are overweight do not feel comfortable being in front of other people in our swimming costumes. By not being able to swim until our middle age makes us feel embarrassed and self-conscious in front of teenagers who are already good swimmers.

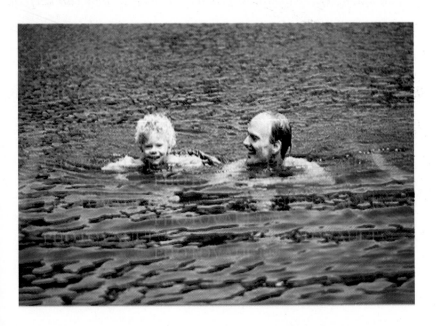

Jogging/ Running

Running is by definition the fastest means for an animal to move on foot. It is defined in sporting terms as a gait in which at some point all feet are off the ground at the same time. It is a form of aerobic exercise.

Mostly athletes are the skinniest people of all the sports players. Still I would not consider many of them skinny, and yet for how long can they stay in such good shape, most probably as long as they can keep on practising. All the big players at some stage in their lives have got to give up and eventually start piling on the pounds.

Is it a good idea to be jumping and running on the road? Yes, if you can find a nice park to run around.

Walking

Energy used in walking 3kilo meter/hr is only 3.7k-cal/ minute. Increase in exercise plays a small part in losing weight.

Any discrepancy in energy balance is important. Obese people use more energy during physical activity but obese people tend to move less.

Cycling

Cycling is a very good exercise and a cheap method of transport. As far as its health properties are concerned, it is a much better idea to pedal instead of travelling by a local bus or train. But you have to take a chance with the weather, and it's not such a good idea if you are wearing a suit and tie on a rainy day. If you are given the choice to buy either a bike or food, definitely you are going to choose food.

Can you really afford to buy a bike and, if you are, when you are going to ride it? The best idea is to use it as a form of transport, it will pay for itself and you will get free exercise.

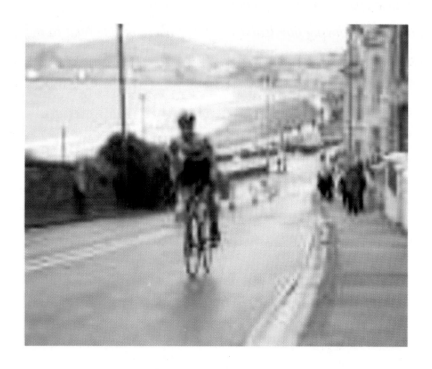

Housework

Housework is not so much an exercise as a routine, yet it is better to do it yourself than to pay and get it done by others. It's also better than sitting on a sofa piling on more pounds.

Life saving drugs

Salt

Healthy 19 to 50-year-old adults should consume 3.8 grams of salt - to replace the amount lost on a daily average through sweat, and to achieve a diet that provides sufficient amounts of other essential nutrients. To replace the body fluids we need a mixture of water and salt in medical terms normal saline.

Water

General recommendations of water consumption for women is approximately 2.7 litres of total water each day and men an average of approximately 3.7 litres. The vast majority of healthy people adequately meet their daily hydration needs by letting thirst be their guide.

Sugar

Sugar is the only food, which we need. Sugar is the only food, which can be consumed by the brain, the only food that transforms into energy.

These three are absolute necessities of life:

Air, water and food

Air

Air is a mixture of gases, including oxygen, which are required for breathing. 100% oxygen is as bad as no oxygen.

Water

Liquid water is the most extraordinary substance. Although we drink it, wash, fish and swim in it, and cook with it, we nearly always overlook the special relationship it has with our lives. Droughts cause famines and floods cause death and disease. It has importance as a solvent, a solute, a reactant and a biomolecule, structuring proteins, nucleic acids and cells. Life cannot evolve or continue without liquid water, which is why there is so much fuss about finding water on Mars, other planets and the moon. It is unsurprising that it plays a central role in many of the world's religions.

The only drink we have on the earth is water.

Water comprises 50 to 70 per cent of an adult's total body weight, and without regular top-ups, our body's survival time is limited to a matter of hours or days.

An inactive person needs between 4-5 pints (2.5 litres) every day to

replace water lost through exhalation, human waste and sweat. In the summer, and during exercise, you will need more than this basic amount, which also varies according to the size of your body.

Water is lost from the body through urine and sweat, and must be replaced through our diets. Chronic dehydration can contribute to a number of health problems, such as constipation and kidney stones.

Drinking plain water is still the most effective way of replacing lost fluids.

The drinking water available from our taps is perfectly adequate to replenish our fluid loss, and undergoes many processes to bring it up to the standards set out in the Water Supply Regulations.

There are certainly no proven health benefits of bottled water over tap water - it basically comes down to personal taste and cost.

An amazing drink, it has been on the earth even before the production of human beings. It is the second cheapest substance to air and has its own taste. By adding other things you just spoil its taste.

Water is the major ingredient of all drinks: carbonated and still drinks are 65% water, diluted squashes are 86% water (after dilution) and fruit juices are 90% water.

Food

No food is 'better for us' than any other.

You should not compare foods with others. Different types of food have different aims. But in the end all foods are going to be processed in the stomach, changing into proteins, carbs and fat from which only glucose is converted into energy and the rest preserved as fat. Only the quantity of food should be considered, appetising-looking food and taste will encourage us to eat more. It does not matter where your food on your plate has been presented to you. Whether it's a 5 star hotel, a well named restaurant or cooked in your own kitchen. The fact of the matter is no food is better than any other in comparison.

It does not matter if you eat proteins, fat or carbohydrates, it is still going to be converted into sugar by the body and then converted into energy. Some of the good material is going to be used to preserve the structure of the body. The rest will be preserved as fat as a preserved source.

Sugar

Sugar is devastating to our health.

One reason is that it is a pure chemical and is the end result of a refining process by which it has been stripped of all the natural nutrition it originally had in the plant itself. Sugar is deleterious to your health: it is more damaging than all other narcotics combined. It is a long-term chemical poison.
Just what damage does sugar do to the human body?

When we talk about sugar, we are including bad nutrition as a whole, since anyone who indulges in sugar has bad dietary habits per se. Sugar is by far the leading cause of dental deterioration - cavities in teeth, bleeding gums, failure of bone structure, and loss of teeth.

Sugar is the main cause of diabetes, hyperglycemias and hypoglycaemias.

It is a significant and a contributory cause of heart disease, arteriosclerosis, mental illness, depression, senility, hypertension, and cancer. The list is endless.

It has an extremely harmful effect in unbalancing the endocrine system and injuring its component glands such as the adrenal glands, pancreas and liver, causing the blood sugar level to fluctuate widely. It has a number of other extremely damaging effects on the human body.

Some of the bad effects of Sugar

- *Increases overgrowth of Candida yeast organism*
- *Increases chronic fatigue*
- *Can trigger binge eating in those with bulimia*
- *Increases PMS symptoms*
- *Increases hyperactivity in about 50% of children*
- *Increases tooth decay*
- *Increases anxiety and irritability*
- *Can increase or intensify symptoms of anxiety and panic in susceptible women*
- *Can make it difficult to lose weight because of constantly high insulin levels, which causes the body to store excess carbohydrates as fat.*

Herbivorous /carnivorous

We are not 'natural carnivores'.

Our jaws do not project forward from the face as they do with cats and dogs. Our front teeth are well adapted for biting fruit and cutting up vegetables.

Our gastric juices contain less hydrochloric acid than carnivores, but are well adapted for the digestion of starches. Our longer colon is suited to a slow process of digestion, extracting a great variety of essential nutrients.

In a sense we are not pure herbivorous either because we cannot digest foods like grass and hay.

What we eat affects not only our own bodies and minds, but also the vast proliferation of humans on the globe. What we eat has a great impact on the whole of the earth.

Meat

I have to talk about meat. I am sorry if that is against your religion, yet what I am talking about is not directed at religion. Most of us abstain from eating meat because of religious reasons, or our teachers said, or as a constitutional document which always does not register in our mind. We should not eat meat because we are humans. Even animals do not eat meat.

Let's talk about animals. Lions eat meat everyone knows that. He kills the animal and he eats the soft parts of the abdomen, which is a half digested, soft vegetarian material. What is left over is eaten by other animals like wolves.

Crocodiles and vultures are some the animals that eat meat, which are ugly looking, lazy animals. The human race was produced as a vegetarian generation. Yet there is a primeval response in our brain that tells us it is acceptable to eat meat in times of emergency, when we do not have anything else to eat and it is a matter of survival, for example in natural disasters. Trust me, at such times humans can even eat the meat of their dead colleagues. There are few examples in the history.

I was talking about Homosapiens.

Charles Darwin says that our ancestors are monkeys and they do not eat meat.

Still I agree with Charles Darwin. Our grand father is a chimpanzee. He eats all fruit and vegetables. He only eats meat when he does not have anything else to eat.

Does meat give you more energy and body building material? Yet where does all the meat from the animal come from, if not from the grass it eats? I had to talk about meat because I have known some people who lived their lives as strict vegetarians, but their death wish was to eat meat because they were restricted to eating meat by religious beliefs, but in their subconscious mind meat was something important but which they were forbidden to eat.

People who were usually meat eaters and who suddenly become vegetarians only because they change religion, cannot be satisfied with just eating vegetarian food because their minds and bodies are tuned into non vegetarian food. And they try to eat something else so in fact they eat more and put on weight.

When you eat meat, do you not think that it was once alive, like you? Someone has killed that animal only to make money and brainwashed you into eating something, which you think is an item of luxury. How can someone's death be another's luxury?

We are animal loving society. We raise chickens, sheep and pigs in our farms. When we go to feed them they come running around us as if they think we are their only saviour, when in fact one day we are going to betray their trust and slaughter them.

I am not trying to make you all vegetarians. As I promised, I have given you the facts, but I am keeping my promise that you can eat what you want to eat when you want to eat.

I will not advise you to eat meat; you can only eat when you have to eat. The medicine textbook says that our main source of fat is meat. Why then doesn't any doctor advise the government to stop trading in meat? The medicine textbook says that you can eat lean meat and white meat. Yet the fat comes from every part of the meat. If we know this is one cause of a heart attack, then why do we eat meat? Anyway my aim is not to make you vegetarian - you can eat whatever you like.

Diseases spread by meat and meat products

Apart from the latest outbreaks of BSE and bird flu, there are many diseases, which do not find their way into the newspapers. Food poisoning by some bacteria and viruses, which proliferate on meat and produce toxins, are ingested with the meat and can make a person seriously ill and can be fatal. There are many other serious diseases like

BSE (Bovine spongiform encephalopathy)

Transmission can occur when healthy animals consume contaminated tissues with TSE proteins

from others with the disease. In the brain it form dense plaque fibers, leading to the microscopic

appearance of "holes" in the brain, degeneration of physical and mental abilities, and ultimately

death. Some TSE's are resistant to extreme temperatures and are not affected by household disinfectants.

Bird flu

Avian influenza (or 'bird flu') is a highly infectious disease affecting many species of

birds, including chickens, duck, turkeys and pet birds. Avian flu passes from birds to other birds,

But there have also been human cases. Avian flu can causes mild symptoms of flu. Some times can

Lead to rapid deterioration, pneumonia and multiple organ failure, which can be fatal.

Breast milk

Breast milk is the primary and best food of our life. That was the only food, which gave us the energy in the first few weeks of our life, and immunity against many diseases for the rest of our life. It is natural, free and gives a bond of love to child and mother. Breast milk is provided by nature and advised by doctors, parents and nurses, and I have never known any one to be against breast-feeding.

Unfortunately not all mothers do breast-feed, and some of the situations when women cannot breast-feed are due to illness.

There are some bad things that can be transmitted to the baby from the

mother. Previously, if the mother had tuberculosis, babies used to be taken away from their mother. In today's society, AIDS is one of the situations when breast-feeding is not advisable. Medicines taken by a mother can also be transmitted to the baby and can produce adverse effects. A usual example is tetracycline in pregnancy and breastfeeding.

When a mother cannot breast feed, or the mother's milk is not enough for that baby, we have to find alternatives. Best is cow's milk, although some people think that goat's milk is lighter than cow's milk. Water can always be added in cow's milk to make it lighter. Nowadays we have

formula milk, which comes in tins. This milk is made according to the requirements of the baby, i.e. the weight and age of the baby. Formula milk is tried, tested and sterilised. Instructions on how to prepare the feed are on the tin.

Milk

What about cow's milk? Has anyone tested that milk today? Was that cow checked for any disease?

You are going to say that milk is pasteurised. The milk in advanced countries arrives in the shops already pasteurised; the rest of the world still relies on boiling the milk. Tell me, is that the only method of sterilising milk? If we do not have enough money to spend on human beings, do we have enough money to spend on animals' health and research? How many diseases are known to be transmitted to humans from dairy products? Only a few.

I disagree with the idea that we only become aware of these diseases after experiencing them.

We did not have AIDS 20 years ago. Likewise, other unknown illness can arrive. We should be putting money into research as a priority, unfortunately that priority cannot be animals. In advanced countries, milk comes from dairy farms where many cows are kept altogether in one place. They are fed mostly on artificial food, and not on grass as we would believe. Their artificial food is treated with many chemicals to aid the production of more milk. Usually animals are treated with antibiotics and steroids, which it is well known are excreted in milk, and therefore enter the food chain.

The cow's body produces this milk. So the milk has the same fat as beef.

We keep the milk in a fridge otherwise it goes off and smells horrible.

Milk is everywhere and forms a part of every one's diet, even in the third world. But not every household is lucky enough to possess a fridge.

The most significant connection between milk and ill health is probably through its contribution to heart disease. Too much saturated fat in the diet can lead to atherosclerosis, where the arteries 'fur up' with cholesterol deposits and cannot deliver enough blood to the vital organs. The heart is particularly susceptible. Milk and other dairy products account for about half of all saturated fats eaten in this country. Meat accounts for the rest.

Dairy products

If we add some yoghurt in the milk and keep it in a warm place overnight, the next day it would have a thick curd, and you might say it smells lovely and tastes nice. In fact the milk has gone off and has the same constituents as rotten milk.

Then process that yoghurt in the food processor and separate the butter and liquid. We keep the butter and throw the liquid away. The liquid, which is the most important constituent of milk, was once a favourite drink of poor farming communities in India who did not have the facilities of milk. It was called lassi. The rich people used to give it to poor people after making butter. That butter used to be preserved by the wealthy people in the village and sold. The more butter in the house means the more well off you are. Milk and milk products are a blessing in those parts of the world. When they can afford it, the first thing they buy is a cow, and if they do not buy a cow then they will buy milk as much as they can. And then they consume that butter which is called desi ghee.

In third world countries, where meat is scarce and cows are sacred, milk and milk products are the main source of fat.

In advanced countries the liquid part is thrown away and the solid part is kept as cheese, which is cassiene and fat. Thought to be tasty, in fact it is rotten milk with some preservatives.

If a medicine textbook says that our main source of fat is meat and

Dairy products, then why do we eat them?

Then that book says we should have skimmed milk, yet if you take all the fat out it would not be called milk. The usual question people ask me in my seminars is where, therefore, would the calcium then come from? The simple answer is, where do the teeth of an elephant come from if he is not drinking cow's milk? And where does the cow itself get milk from? Of course it is all green leafy grass.

It is my opinion that if dairy products did not exist, the mortality and morbidity rate from heart disease would reduce down to fifty percent.

Diseases transmitted through milk

Most children who are bottle-fed feel sick due to the contamination of milk during the preparation process, causing diarrhoea, vomiting and fever and leads to dehydration and malnutrition. Cattle, buffalo and bison, are the natural host of M. bovis. Bovine tuberculosis is well known to be transmitted through milk. Hepatitis A, Salmonella and Shigela can be transmitted through contaminated milk. AIDS is the most concerned disease, and at this time there is no cure. Breast-feeding is considered to be a possible method of transmission of AIDS.

Farming Animals

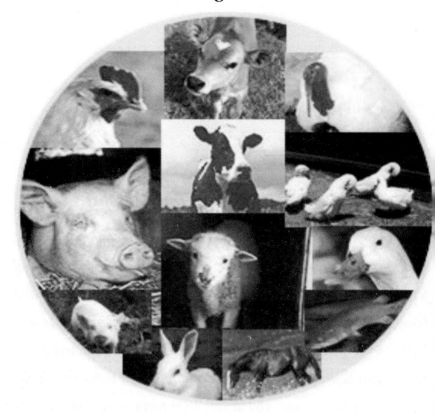

Pigs

There are around 7-8 million pigs in the UK, reared primarily for bacon, ham, pork and sausages. Pigs are naturally intelligent and inquisitive social animals. Originally pigs lived in woodlands, foraging for nuts, seeds, roots and grubs. They will not soil their resting area and the myth that pigs are somehow dirty comes from their wallowing in wet mud. They do this to cool down in hot weather and to rid themselves of pests.

Cows

Cow's milk is a liquid secreted by the mammary glands of the adult female cow to nourish her young calf until weaned. Before the cow can produce milk, in common with other species of mammal, she must first become pregnant and give birth.

Cows are sacred in Indian communities due to many reasons. They provide a living to millions of people, mainly by milk and ploughing by bulls. They are prayed to, and have a high spiritualistic value equal to gods. They are never slaughtered, and eating beef is against the Indian religion.

In the modern world, in comparison, every part of the animal is used, meat as well as dairy products. It is a big industry.
Poultry

Lean chicken has the same amount of cholesterol as lean beef. All muscle meat has far too much cholesterol, protein and fat, even if you can't see it. The protein in chicken is just as bad for you as the protein in beef, because your body has to work so hard to get rid of it. Chicken is just as bad for you as beef or lamb.

Eggs

Eggs contain cholesterol and high cholesterol levels in our blood increases our risk of heart disease. Assuming one egg contains 200 mg cholesterol, consuming one egg a day increases the total cholesterol by 0.111 m mol /L, increasing the risk of myocardial infarction by an estimated 2%. Eggs are an animal product for the purpose of regeneration and reproduction. We are interfering in the law of nature and that's why there is a reduction in the number of animals on the earth. That could also be the reason why dinosaurs became extinct, because somehow the reproduction cycle of dinosaurs was halted.

Eating raw eggs causes biotin and pentothenic acid (vitB6) deficiency resulting in dermatitis. If we know that eggs are a source of cholesterol, why we do we eat them? Why stop the regeneration process of some animals?

Bread

In the mill, the grain passes through more than forty processes before it emerges as flour and bran. This is how bread is made.

1 level teaspoon salt
1 level teaspoon sugar
1 level tablespoon soft margarine
1 sachet (6g) easy blend dried yeast or fast action easy blend dried yeast
2/3-cup warm water
1 ½ Cups of flour

Commercial yeast is a by-product of the whisky distillers.

Before we even start baking our bread, there are enough poisons like margarine, salt, sugar and yeast already present in the bread. Yeasts can provoke a number of reactions in some people, particularly skin disorders.

Beware of 'brown bread'. This type of bread is made using refined flour with an added agent such as caramel to give it its brown colour it's nothing to do with fibre. It doesn't have any of the goodness of the grain.

Wholemeal bread is made from the flour, which is not sieved, and thus it has the main constituents of grain; wholemeal dough is not easy to knead and that's why it costs more.

Carbohydrates

All carbohydrates are digested in the body to form glucose, which is transported around the body via the blood and taken into cells to be converted into energy. The hormone insulin, secreted by the pancreas gland within the abdomen, controls this action of cell glucose uptake.

Excess glucose is converted into glycogen, which is stored in the liver or in fat around the body. If the body needs more energy, a second hormone, glucagons, is secreted by the pancreas, which converts the glycogen back into glucose. It is then released back into the bloodstream so that, with the help of the insulin, the cells can take up the glucose to release the energy they need.

As you can see, the glucose or sugar metabolism of the body is a cycle of glucose, insulin and glucagons reactions. The slower the release of glucose and hormones, the more stable and sustainable the energy levels of the body. It is generally accepted that the more refined the carbohydrate, the faster the glucose is released into the blood and the less stable the energy levels of the body.

The complex carbohydrates provide a slower and more sustained release of energy than the simple carbohydrates. For long-term good health, appetite control and sustained energy levels, unrefined complex carbohydrates are recommended as part of our daily diet.

Apparently, carbohydrates were extremely important, even more than protein. Government studies into carbohydrates show that we all need a lot of carbohydrates every day. Do not believe that we all need 1000's of grams of carbohydrates every day.

Grain is the main staple diet of all the population on earth. Wheat is the main source of carbohydrates; potatoes, maize and rice are others. Wheat can be grown almost anywhere in the world.

Human consumption of corn constitutes a staple food in many regions of the world. Corn meal is made into a thick porridge in many cultures. Sweet corn is a high in sugars and low in starch that is served like a vegetable. Popcorn is kernels of certain varieties that explode when heated, forming fluffy pieces that are eaten as a snack.

Polenta is a gluten free, low fat and high carbohydrate diet.

Fats

Fats provide a concentrated source of energy in the diet. These can be either saturated, monounsaturated or poly-unsaturated. Foods rich in saturated fats are usually of animal origin. Vegetable fats are generally unsaturated.

Saturated fat raises the level of cholesterol in the blood. Cholesterol is present in animal foods but not plant foods.

Fats and oils are essentially the same. Fats tend to be solid at room temperature whilst oils are liquid. The medicine textbook says that there is no necessity for a dietary intake of fats.

Essential fatty acids can be synthesized in the body; therefore dietary supply is not essential.

Even in low fat diets subcutaneous fat storage can be normal.

Fatty acid deficiency is only seen in people who are in hospital for parenteral nutrition with proteins and glucose.

Saturated fat (animal fat) and some vegetable oils, e.g., coconut, palm oil, increase the risk of cholesterol. This causes narrowing or furring of the arteries and increases the risk of a heart attack or stroke.

Eating saturated fats increases the amount of LDL cholesterol in your blood. In some foods saturated fat is easy to see, e.g., the fat on meat and cream on a pint of whole milk. However, much of the saturated fat that we eat is hidden in processed foods

Gluten

Gluten is an amorphous protein combined with starch in some cereals, wheat, rye and barley. It constitutes about 80% of the proteins contained in wheat. Gluten is responsible for the elasticity of kneaded dough. Some people can not tolerate gluten, a condition called Coeliac Disease. Around 1 in 1000 people are affected by this condition. This is intolerance to gluten, a protein found in wheat.

Proteins

Proteins make up about 15% of the mass of the average person. Much of the fabric of our body is constructed from protein molecules. Muscle, cartilage, ligaments, skin and hair - these are all mainly protein materials.

In addition to these large-scale structures that hold us together, other proteins play a vital role in keeping our body working properly such as haemoglobin, hormones (such as insulin), anti bodies and enzymes.

Our bodies are unable to store extra protein. Unfortunately extra protein is converted to and stored as fat.

In athletes, consuming excess protein can seriously affect their ability to train and compete at peak performance.

Excess protein may lead to dehydration, ketosis (high levels of blood acids), potassium and calcium depletion, muscle weakness and possible kidney problem.

Vitamins

Vitamin B complex and vitamin C are water-soluble vitamins and are found in fruit and vegetables. Vitamin B12, which is not found in Vegan food, is found in sufficient quantities if you are an occasional meat eater. Or use occasional dairy products.

Contrary to popular belief, vegetarians suffer no more from anaemia than do meat-eaters.

Other good sources of folic acid, other than meats, are asparagus, Brussels sprouts, spinach, romaine lettuce, collard greens, and broccoli. Other good sources are black-eyed peas, cantaloupe, orange, oatmeal, whole grain cereals, and wheat germ.

Eat fresh, raw fruits and vegetables often. Don't overcook food. Heat destroys folic acid. Supplementation with maternal folic acid alone had no affect on birth size.

The causes of vitamin deficiencies need to be identified and treated. There is no need to supply vitamins to the body unnecessarily. Good sources of vitamin B12 for vegetarians are dairy products or free-range eggs. ½ pint of milk (full fat or semi skimmed) contains 1.2 μg.

A slice of vegetarian cheddar cheese (40g) contains 0.5 μg. A boiled egg contains 0.7 μg. Fermentation in the manufacture of yoghurt destroys much of the B12 present. Boiling milk can also destroy much of the B12.

Vegans are recommended to ensure their diet includes foods fortified with vitamin B12. A range of B12 fortified foods are available. These include yeast extracts, Soya milks, vegetable and sunflower margarines, and breakfast cereals.

Supplements

Vitamins cannot be separated and kept in raw form, they have to be processed and separated and prepared in chemical formulae by the pharmaceutical companies. Most of them have chemical constituents for preservation and a basic component to keep them in powder liquid or solid form. Why do we have these chemicals without any reason, unless we are suffering from any illness? If you have any problem like Malabsorption Syndrome or g6pd deficiency syndrome, you should be in regular contact with your doctor. Do not take any vitamin supplement.

The usual cause of B12 deficiency is not a lack of it in the diet but the inability to absorb it from food.

Vitamin D and A

Vitamin D is a fat-soluble vitamin, which acts like a hormone, regulating the formation of bone and the absorption of calcium and phosphorus from the intestine. It helps to control the movement of calcium between bone and blood, and vice versa. The most significant supply of vitamin D comes from the action of ultra-violet B light on sterols in the skin.

Vitamin A helps in the growth and repair of body tissues, especially bones, and the formation and maintenance of tooth enamel and gums and night vision.

We can obtain a sufficient supply of vitamin A from carrots, apricots, sweet potatoes, dandelion greens, spinach, cantaloupe, oat flakes, and raisin bran, so we do not have to include beef, liver, swordfish and butter in our diet.

Minerals

Calcium, magnesium

Magnesium is a constituent of chlorophyll and so is widely available in green leafy vegetables and it is also available in cereals.

Good sources of calcium include green leafy vegetables, seeds and nuts - which contain more than four times the calcium of whole cow's milk. Calcium in green leafy vegetables is absorbed better than the calcium from cow's milk. Drinking hard water can provide 200mg of calcium daily but soft water contains almost none. Other calcium rich foods include black molasses, edible seaweeds, watercress, parsley and dried figs.

Fibre

I am very keen on a high fibre diet. Not only is it the most natural, convenient and healthy way to look after our bodies, but fibre helps to control weight by satisfying hunger and helping you to feel full for much longer

Nuts, seeds and pulses are all rich in fibre. But as with all cereal foods, like bread, pasta and rice, the amount of fibre depends on how they were processed. The outer layer of grain is removed during refining and with it, much of the vitamins and minerals.

Fruit and vegetable juices also work; especially prune juice and apple-pear juice, which is particularly laxative. Adding one gram of fibre adds five grams of bulk in your stools.

Try not to use a juicing machine as they usually discard the fibre and this is precisely the part you need. Juicing machines are only introduced for the old and the ill who cannot eat fruits raw.

Toxins

Snake venom
There are some snakes whose bite is so deadly it can cause death within a matter of seconds. Nevertheless, even snake venom, deadly as it is, has been used for therapeutic, medical purposes when used in minute quantities.

Nicotine

Nicotine is as poisonous as snake venom.

Nicotine is a stimulant drug, but paradoxically its effects are both stimulation and relaxation. The addictive effect of nicotine is linked to its capacity to trigger the release of dopamine - a chemical in the brain that is associated with feelings of pleasure. However, recent research has suggested that in the long term, nicotine depresses the ability of the brain to experience pleasure. Thus, smokers need greater amounts of the drug to achieve the same levels of satisfaction. Smoking is therefore a form of self-medication: further smoking alleviates the withdrawal symptoms, which set in soon after the effects.

If you are a smoker, being overweight is not your problem. Your problem is smoking.

Smoking adds to the problems of overweight people, not the other way round. Get some help and give up that filthy disgusting habit! It is much easier to cut down weight than to give up smoking. Do not even think that if you stop smoking you will put some weight on. Even if you do put extra weight on, it can be sorted out later, but not the other way round. Young girls think that smoking keeps their weight down, but in fact when people become addicted to smoking they either smoke or eat more to try to stop chain smoking, which results in obesity.

Coffee and Tea

Caffeine is the main constituent of coffee and tea.

Caffeine is an alkaloid, which is a compound found in cola nut, cacao beans, tea and other plants.

Caffeine is present in different amounts according to the different plant sources.

Caffeine stimulates the central nervous system, heart muscle and respiratory system. It has diuretic effects (increased urine) and delays fatigue and increases alertness.

Caffeine has been used as a weight-loss aid in the past because of its ability to improve metabolism. But it has not been used for this purpose for many years because there is no evidence that it helps people to lose weight.

Caffeine is also used in combination with painkillers such as aspirin to provide headache relief, but there is little evidence for its use for this purpose.

High intake of caffeine at once can cause caffeine-induced mental disorder. The symptoms include restlessness, nervousness, excitement, insomnia, stomach upset, muscle twitching, incoherent speech, heart palpitations and excessive alertness.

Even at much lower doses, too much caffeine can have unwanted side effects.

Coffee consumption can cause a rise in blood pressure for a few hours in people sensitive to the effects of caffeine.

Large caffeine consumption in the elderly has been linked to an increased risk of hip fracture and loss of bone density.

It may also aggravate the effects of irritable bowel syndrome.
High coffee consumption has also been linked to problems in pregnancy. Caffeine has caused birth defects in rats. There is strong evidence that caffeine may reduce a baby's birth weight. Caffeine has also been shown to reduce sperm movement.

Withdrawal effects

Caffeine withdrawal can produce several side effects. These include:

Headaches, Irritability, Nervousness, Restlessness and Tiredness

Caffeine amounts in popular soft drinks per 12 oz cans:

Coca-Cola/45.6mgs
Diet-Cola/45.6mgs

Have you ever eaten coffee? Have you ever tasted coffee?

If not get a teaspoonful and put it on your tongue - you will not be able to swallow it. Rather you will throw up and run towards the tap to wash it off and will feel horrible for hours afterwards.

That black-brown powder, which does not look good and tastes horrible, is diluted thousands of times into a mug and yet still you cannot drink it. Then you add some milk, but still it does not taste good and you put some sugar in it. Still it does not taste good and you add

some cream and sprinkle some chocolate on it and give it a fancy name called cappuccino.

Why go to such effort to swallow a horrible disgusting brown powder and then get addicted to it?

You do not need it. It does not have any ingredient, which is beneficial to you, rather you have added milk, sugar and chocolate, which are all dangerous to your health.

Salt

Is it the cheapest and most important food ingredient available on earth? It caused the demise of British rule in India.

Since 75% of the salt we eat comes from everyday foods, such as some breakfast cereals, soups, sauces, ready meals and biscuits, it's easy to eat too much salt without adding any yourself. In fact, one or two servings of some foods could contain more than your daily limit of salt (1g). Salt retains one litre of the water in your body which results in hypertension and heart failure.

Soda bicarbonate

Soda bicarbonate is alkaline in nature. It is used for therapeutic purposes in highly titrated doses. It is used in baking as a raising agent. It gives a light open texture to cakes and scones, and is used as a substitute for yeast in making soda bread. Sodium bicarbonate is actually a cleaning agent. Having such a strong chemical agent added in your food I do not think is a clever idea.

Chocolate

Chocolate is made from cocoa beans, which are fermented, roasted and mixed with alkali to make it solid. Dark chocolate is made by combining chocolate liquor with sugar, cocoa butter, and vanilla. To make milk chocolate, chocolate liquor is combined with cocoa butter, sugar, and milk solids or powder. White chocolate is made without chocolate liquor. It is the cocoa butter that gives it the chocolate flavour. Dipping chocolate is made with more cocoa butter than regular eating chocolate.

Chocolate is addictive. Research suggested that people who eat too much chocolate have a lower life expectancy. Chocolate's high fat content means that excess indulgence can contribute to obesity, leading to an increased risk of heart disease.

Soft Drink

The recent scare of pesticides found in soft drink bottles in India is not news. Hyperactivity syndrome in children is associated with soft drinks. Most of the soft drinks are addictive. Drinking diet brands does not take the addictive factor out. All of them cause diuresis leading further to dehydration.

Alcohol

If you are drinking more than 50 units a week you are likely to have physical, mental and social problems. Even though I have never stopped any one from drinking alcohol, here are some facts.

Even though there is no fat as such in a pint of lager, there are however about 180 calories of energy.

Alcohol is a poison that can cause irreversible damage to the liver.

Heavy drinking is blamed for up to 33,000 deaths a year in the UK. In Britain nearly one in ten men and one in twenty women have an alcohol problem.

Drinkers are more likely to have casual sex that leads to unwanted pregnancies and sexually transmitted diseases.

Alcohol is estimated to be the cause of about 2030 % of road traffic accidents.

Even in low quantities, long-term alcoholics suffer from Myopathies, which reduce in physical activity and bone deformities.

Alcohol in pregnancy, even in small quantities, causes small babies.

Food and alcohol has been a combination for centuries. It means that we are adding to the calorific value of food, which we are trying to cut down.

Food, which is often eaten with alcohol, is meat, fish and crisps and a salty nut, which makes us thirstier and leads us to drink more and add to our food problems Spirits are bitter in taste and increase our appetite. We add soda, juice or cola to make the taste palatable, which adds to the bad effects of food.

Fruits and vegetables

Delicious crunchy apples, sweet strawberries, juicy peaches and exotic juices make your mouth water by just thinking about them. Fresh fruit always makes a tasty and nutritious snack.
Fruit and vegetables can help keep your body fitter, healthier and happier. They are packed with vitamins and minerals.

They can help you to maintain a healthy weight. They're an excellent source of fibre and antioxidants. They help reduce the risk of heart disease, stroke and some cancers.

They taste delicious and there's so much variety to choose from. Fruit and vegetables in the diet have many positive effects upon health. Their high dietary fibre content helps control blood glucose levels, reduces blood cholesterol and probably reduces the risk of cancers.
They contain not only antioxidants but also phytochemicals, which may reduce the risk of coronary heart disease. More than any other foods, they contain essential vitamins such as A, B, C, E and folic acid and minerals like potassium, calcium, zinc and manganese, which are all vital for good health and disease prevention.
Fruit juices lose most of their natural fibre in the juicing process.

Dried fruits

With its sweet or sharp flavours and chewy or fleshy textures, dried fruit can be eaten any time of the day; as a breakfast cereal, a lunchtime salad, or adding a bite to a dinner dish. Dried fruits can be used to make a tasty sauce, mixed, chopped. They even make a healthy snack - an alternative natural sweetener full of vitamins and minerals food.

Asian food

Indian food and Chinese restaurants

Today it is impossible to imagine a high street in the UK without an Indian restaurant offering curry. But the Indian restaurants are not really Indian. To have such a wide choice of foods one would have to travel thousands of miles in India. 80% of people of India are living below the poverty line. This means they can only afford their one basic meal a day. Normally they cannot afford butter and meat, which are the most expensive items in the Indian meal. That's why starving people do not suffer from heart illnesses.

Salt is the main poison in Asian foods. When making meat curries we retain all the fat in the curry.
In Britain, Asian food is made richer by adding cheese, butter, colouring agents and more spices.

In the modern India majority of people do not die of starvation. The wells to do Indian people have a high mortality and morbidity rate from diabetes and heart diseases because of their food made rich with meat and dairy products.

Italian pizza and pastas

Pizzas and pasta is the Italian staple diet. Problems occur when they are mixed with meat, cheese and other food additives for the toppings.
Fish and chips

We put batter on the fish, which is a carbohydrate. Then we fry the fish, which takes out all the moisture, essential fatty acids and vitamins. The remaining fish is tasteless and odourless. The excess oil starts smelling of fish, it is not reusable and is difficult to dispose off.

Potatoes are the main source of carbohydrates. When we peel them we lose some of the essential nutrients of potatoes. Then we fry them, which takes out the moisture and cover them with oil.

Carbohydrates are alkaline in nature. Proteins are acidic in nature, which together makes a neutral mass, which is no good to our body. Rather, it is more work for the body to expel it.

Vinegar

Vinegar is a clear liquid, consisting chiefly of acetic acid, obtained by the fermentation of wine, cider or malt beer. It is used to flavour food and is a preservative in pickling.

It is actually a cleaning agent.

Fast food chains

There is no doubt that foods which are high in fat, high in sugar and high in salt are unhealthy.

School meals

For years children in our schools have been eating food, which has proven to be worse than junk food. Children have developed the taste for that food.

Thanks to Jamie Oliver, a celebrity chef, for introducing awareness of food in schools. Now schools are thinking of changing their menu to introduce more healthy choices. I hope they do not introduce the same meals as those offered to NHS patients.

Our generation has a tendency to complicate things. If we want to make it simple, why not just park a lorry full of fruit in the school grounds so that the children can eat any fruit at any time during their breaks? That also leaves a choice of home cooked meals at dinnertime.

Diets

There are one hundred and eighteen methods of dieting on the market at this time, and nearly every one is as effective as the other.

High street superstores know that most of the people are turning against the food they sell, so they have decided to introduce their own diet foods. They do not taste like the original food, yet the cost has definitely gone up. The cheaper food that you can buy from the high street is high in fat, salt and sugar. The result is that people who cannot afford to buy the more expensive, healthy food are likely to get fat and ill.

Weight reducing medicine

Most of the weight reducing medicines on the market are dangerous and contain addictive chemicals. They are meant for something else, and weight reduction is only their side effect. Drugs may help people to lose weight, but the problem is keeping it off. Most people who lose weight on a calorie controlled diet put it on again. Only 5% of obese people manage to keep their weight down.

Food allergy

As in Peanut anaphylaxis - where we have an immediate catastrophic reaction a food allergy will require emergency adrenaline injections and medical resuscitation.

Food Intolerance, which may be due to enzyme deficiencies and other mechanisms that mimic true allergic reactions. Some cause diarrhoea, vomiting and heartburns. Sometimes people have headaches, muscle and joint aches and pains, and tiredness.

Many foods and food products can provoke allergic reactions.

Food additives, particularly tartrazine and sodium benzoate, can provoke urticaria, rhinitis and asthma. Yeasts can provoke a number of reactions in some people, particularly skin disorders. There are many colouring agents used for food to look good. Most of them are suspected to cause cancer.

Food preservatives

When storing foods, preservatives are used to ensure that the condition of the foods remain stable, fresh and retain vitamin and minerals. Some of them are:

Sulphur dioxide, salt and vinegar, benzoates and sorbates.

These are found most frequently in processed meats, drinks, meats, salads, margarines, jams, cheeses and pickled foods.

By adding food preservatives we not only change the taste of the food but also destroy some of the important constituents of the food.

Detox remedies

There are many detox remedies available in the market.

Why waste time and money to detoxify your body when you have a simple formula available at home?

Do not take more toxins than your body can handle. Drink plenty of water. It's a solute, which dissolves the toxins and takes them out through urine and other excretory systems. It is a natural cleanser which nature has provided us.

Plastic surgery

This is the modern age when we can use our clinicians, who are supposed to help the ailing. Nowadays they can help you to look the way you want to be. Apart from plastic surgery being expensive, it has plenty of health risks. The main risks are that you might not achieve what you are looking for. The other is that it can have the reverse effect and, worse, it can endanger your life. Whether you decide to have liposuctions or the bats removed under your arms, the general risks will be the same.

All surgery carries some uncertainty and risk, including the possibility of infection, bleeding, blood clots, and adverse reactions to the anaesthesia. You may find it hard to stand up straight after a tummy tuck operation and it will feel as if your stomach is tugging. You may also experience numbness in the area treated for liposuction and the scars will be permanent.

A tummy tuck and liposuction will not stop you gaining weight in the future. A tummy tuck operation should be only used to remove excess skin after you have reached your ideal shape and size.

Methods of Measurement
Calories and weight

An average man or woman needs 3000 calories when they lead an active lifestyle, like manual workers on farms, construction workers and nursery workers. When they get promoted to become supervisors or work as supervisors they need only 2000 calories. If they carry on consuming 3000 calories they will start putting on weight by 50 grams a day. The process of putting on weight is so slow that you cannot notice it, until or unless you record your weight or compare it to your old photographs.
Overeating by 1000k cal a day can lead to a 10-kilo weight gain in two years.

If I advise overweight people to consume only 2000 calories, according to a strict dieting regime, they will only maintain their weight and cannot cut it down. Really to cut down weight drastically they need to be consuming only 1000 calories a day, which is enough to live on. This would reduce their weight by 50 grams a day, as I explained earlier. In extreme cases even 500 calories a day are enough.

Other methods of measurement I do not like, as they never make sense.

- *Body mass index (BMI)*
- *Basal metabolic rate (BMR)*
- *Surface area (Sq. Meters)*
- *Micrograms (M.grammes)*
- *Joules*
- *Kilojoules (K. joules)*
- *Kcal (Kilos)*

These are very difficult terms to understand by definition. Then you have to understand the use of it. I spent weeks learning about them when I was a medical student because I knew they were important for my patients, and also important for me to know so that I could use them to help my patients. I calculated the calories with a calorimeter when I was at university. I still could not understand how an ordinary person could count the calories in his food and how much he could use during the day. I have not seen any calorimeter on the market to buy.

The method of measurement I want you to adopt is the mirror. Stand up with minimal clothes in front of the mirror every now and then and see the bulges and curves of your body, and ask yourself is that the way you want to be, or do you want to do some thing about it?

The second method is to take a photograph of yourself today, compare it with old photos and keep a record of when, where and how they were taken.

Some definitions

Diarrhoea - loose stools

Stomach pains, feeling sick and vomiting, often accompany diarrhoea. It is usually due to consumption of drinking water contaminated with bacteria, undercooked meat and eggs or inadequate kitchen hygiene - in other words, an infection. In diarrhoea, dehydration proceeds immediately to a threatening situation.

Steatorrhoea

Steatorrhoea is an excess of fat in faeces. The stool may float due to trapped air.

Constipation

Difficulty in the passage of stools
There are two main causes of Constipation: inactive lifestyle and insufficient fluid intake. Constipation is the main cause of painful conditions like piles and fissure in ano.

Vomiting

Vomiting is a forceful ejection of gastric juice due to inflammation of the stomach, usually by the result of infection by bacteria or virus. There is not much a doctor can do about it. Vomiting usually accompanies diarrhoea. The main danger is dehydration, and it is better to replace the fluids by continuous sipping of isotonic water.

Hiccups

Involuntary diaphragmatic contractions may occur after a large meal, alcohol intake or after excitement.

Dental caries

Dental caries, also known as tooth decay, that damages the structure of teeth. Fermentation of sugars by plaque bacteria causes caries by decalcification of enamel and dentine

Tooth decay usually does not cause symptoms until you have a cavity or an infected tooth. You can easily prevent tooth decay by brushing and flossing your teeth regularly. While eating meat, pieces of flesh get stuck in between the teeth, which get dissolved as acid and cause tooth decay.

Mouth ulcers

A mouth ulcer is a breach or break in the mucous membrane, which lines the inside of the mouth. It may be caused by minor injuries from teeth or food. Mouth ulcers of unknown cause are called aphthous ulcers. They are more likely to occur at times of stress. They may occur after eating certain foods. Usually they heal in a week.

Cold sores

Cold sores are a very common illness caused by the herpes simplex virus.

Halitosis - bad breath

This is usually caused by rotten teeth. If your teeth and gums are in poor health they may be one of the causes of bad breath. Regular, competent dental care is important in controlling bad breath odour. Some of the foods we eat can cause bad breath odour. Garlic, onions, alcohol, hot peppers or aromatic spices may cause bad breath.

Ketosis is a process in which your body converts fats into energy. During the conversion, ketones are produced as a by-product. Ketones can give your breath a sweet, fruity smell that may be mistaken for alcohol.

Flatulence - excessive wind

Some of the wind in the stomach is taken during the process of glutition. The chemical reactions and the normal bacteria in the intestine of the body produce other gases. Passing wind through the mouth and the anus is a normal process, but the wrong type of food can produce foul smelling wind.

Dysphagia

Dysphagia is known as difficulty in swallowing. It usually occurs in illnesses of the oesophagus.

Heartburns

Heartburns are a retrosternal burning pain. The heartburn pain caused by the irritation of the oesophagus is a burning pain which you feel in the centre of the chest. Obesity leads to a higher pressure in the abdomen.

Pregnancy causes a higher pressure in the abdomen and there is also evidence that the changing hormone levels cause relaxation of the muscle valve.

Large amounts of food and drink cause back pressure.

This occurs in gastritis, and stomach ulcers need to be taken serious. Sudden pain in the same area can be serious and can be associated with the heart.

Cancers

Cancers of the lips, mouth, tongue and oesophagus are associated with smoking, while other cancers of the intestinal tract are associated with a low fibre diet.

Diabetes

If you are diabetic and you take insulin, do not change your diet without consulting your doctor. Your insulin dose is titrated against your food intake. Any change in diet can lead to severe hypoglycaemia or hyperglycaemia.

Are you hungry?

These things determine whether you are hungry or not:

1. Timing breakfast time, lunchtime and dinnertime.

2. When you want to eat something. That is an urge triggered by smell, looks and even just by thinking about food.

3. Whether you are thirsty.

4. When you are really hungry, when you really need to eat something, your body is telling you that you cannot go any further because your fuel reserves are depleted.

How we go about it?

We have to change those habits, not for a few days or weeks, but for the rest of our lives. You can start enjoying your life now. The majority of food we eat is not our choice but the result of conditioning from birth. Most of the decisions are made by either the parents or the person who cooks. You cannot go into Gordon Ramsey's kitchen and tell him to cook the food you want and cook it in your way. You know what he is going to say.

Explore yourself

First and foremost, I would advise you to explore yourself. Identify in yourself the way you wish to be, by using your eyes, ears and touch. What are the things you like in yourself and the things you do not like in yourself?

The first method is to look at yourself in a mirror with minimal clothing. Have a proper look at what you like in your body and what you do not like, and ask yourself why.
You can feel the curves and bulges of your body. Do you like your body, if not why? The simple idea is that if you do not like your body, then it's likely someone else will not either. Take a photograph if you feel comfortable enough.

Tell yourself all the things you do and don't like about your body, by speaking out loud.

I have two other experiments.
Stand independently on the floor and put your shoes on and tie the laces without holding on to anything. Weigh yourself and record it. I have provided a form in this book. Fill it in. Keep all the records somewhere safe.

Now is the time to make changes in your eating habits for life. But that's where the catch is: you are not going on a dieting mission, your idea is not just to reduce your weight, your idea is to eat what you like and eat when you like and stay healthy for life. Eating salads and celery soup is not the idea of living life to the full.

Favourite meal (meal 2)

Now is the time when you can enjoy your favourite meal of the day. You have worked hard today to earn that meal and you are hungry enough to enjoy that meal. Have a sip of water, which will make your taste buds clean to feel the exact taste of the meal. Enjoy your meal in small boluses and chew it completely to make it half solid so that it is mixed with the juices of your mouth, which have capabilities to partially digest the food even before swallowing. Try to taste every ingredient in your meal. If you find something more or insufficient in it, you can improve your meal next time. Keep your meal as simple as you can so that you can enjoy each individual taste. If you are cooking a mixture of vegetables and covering them with gravy, you are actually tasting the gravy and not the individual items. A plate of roast vegetables will taste the same as meat. Keep a cup of gravy separate and dip your boluses separately so that you can feel the different tastes. As discussed earlier, try not to eat meat and dairy products.

How much I should eat?

As much as you like.

Portions

Portions of your food are also not decided by you. No one can force-feed you, but you are conditioned as a child to finish the plate because food is expensive, someone had made an effort to cook and you would not like to waste it would you? But it works the other way round, as "matter can neither be created nor be destroyed only it can be transformed into one form to another". Food, which is left over on the plate, can be recycled into compost, which is then consumed by plants to help them to grow.

The food that is over eaten by you not only goes to waste but it will give you health problems, like those discussed earlier. Getting bigger and fatter is not going to help any starving child in India or Africa.

If you have any leftover food today, just leave it and let it go into the compost bin. Next time you will know exactly how much to cook without there being any left over.

When you are finished with your meal today, this is the best time to discuss your favourite meal tomorrow. Again keep it simple. Keep yourself busy and whenever you are not busy think about your meal, what a lovely meal it was and how much better it is going to be tomorrow.

Carry on with this feeding routine for six days.

Starters

Eat one course meal at a time; do not spoil your meal by eating a starter. This way you are destroying your hunger and it will spoil the actual good meal you have been waiting for.

Desserts

Ice creams, yoghurts and coffees sound good but you will not enjoy them because you have fulfilled your appetite; you have enjoyed a perfectly healthy and tasty meal, so why would you want to destroy it by having desert. Most of the desserts are rich in fat, salt and sugar, even a small portion of dessert fills you up, and that you have already done with your favourite meal. Still I am not stopping you from eating your favourite desserts. You can enjoy those things some other day when you are next hungry.

Beverages

I am not in favour of drinking with food. If you are drinking socially within your limits, having a drink with salad enables you to taste the original taste of drink as well. I myself am in favour of a nightcap. One drink at bed time makes me secure in the knowledge that I am drinking within my limit, and keeps me away from drinking and driving, and it helps me to nod off to sleep and thus postpone those worries for tomorrow.

Breakfast, lunch and dinner

We have divided our food into breakfast, dinner and lunch. If we have breakfast, which gives us the fuel we need for the day, then why do we have lunch? Why do we have to have lunch when breakfast was enough to provide us with enough energy for the day, and why do we have our dinner when we do not have any work to do over night? We only do this because we feel hungry. Let me rephrase this, it is only because we want to eat something or we are in the habit of eating lunch and dinner. As soon as I looked at the clock it was 1300. I started feeling hungry, or perhaps I felt hungry after smelling the cooking from the canteen. We are accustomed to eating three meals a day, not because we feel hunger and we need to eat. After decades of medical research, still we have not decided when is the best time to eat and when not to. Why can't we eat when we want to? That is exactly my answer - instead of eating breakfast, dinner or lunch we should eat whenever we want to.

Do not have breakfast.

Do not have lunch.

Do not have dinner.

Eat whenever you want to eat.

Eat whatever you want to eat.

Try eating your vegetables raw.
Microwave or lightly steam your vegetables. These methods retain the

nutrients, and preparation is easy and less time consuming.

Salads are quick to make and can be made more exotic and appetising by adding sliced peppers, cherry tomatoes, beans and a healthy dressing.
Always wash your vegetables before use and remove the outer leaves of lettuces and cabbage.

To gain the maximum benefit from fruit, ensure that whenever possible it is fresh, and if the skins are edible, eat them too.

Combine fruits like oranges and mangos.
Have fresh fruit in your breakfast, lunch and dinner.
Choose dried fruits that have not been preserved.

Exercise

As explained earlier, no exercise alone can reduce your weight, but exercise is absolute necessity as much as your food is. The exercise I am going to advise you today is simple, does not cost anything and is easy to perform. You do not need any equipment for this and I am not going to sell you anything.

Walk

You can walk on the pavement, in the park, school grounds or even in your own garden or wherever is convenient for you. It is better if you can separate your walk from your routine work. You can walk in the morning, in the evening or whenever you can get time; it is better if you can walk every day at the same time. The advantage to this is that, slowly but surely, it becomes a daily routine as well as a habit. Even if you are feeling under the weather, coming out in the fresh air and walking is important. Even disabled people who can not walk, it is important for them to get out by whatever means they have, whether it is a wheelchair, sticks or crutches. After sickness or illness, this is a very good exercise. You can start today and there is no age restriction, even at the oldest age with the help of sticks or crutches. Even bedridden patients need to be exercised passively.

How much one should walk in a day?

There is no restriction, you can walk as much as you want or can. After an illness, if you are learning to walk again take it slowly, walk as much as you can and stop, wait a moment, balance your breath and start again. An average person should walk at least half an hour and children and young adults for an hour. You can take your friend to accompany you, take your family with you or keep a dog as a best friend. You do not need any equipment; you just wear clothes according to the weather.

How much one should walk in a day?

There is no restriction, you can walk as much as you want or can. After an illness, if you are learning to walk again take it slowly, walk as much as you can and stop, wait a moment, balance your breath and start again. An average person should walk at least half an hour and children and young adults for an hour. You can take your friend to accompany you, take your family with you or keep a dog as a best friend. You do not need any equipment; you just wear clothes according to the weather.

Seventh day itch

Now you have been eating according to your new routine for six days. If you have been counting your days, there is no need to, because you have to change your eating habits and you are not on a dieting mission and therefore you have every right to enjoy yourself. If you feel that you have been restricted to any kind of food, or you have restricted yourself, this is the day you can do whatever you like. Keep one day a week. I call it a luxury day, but in fact every day has been a luxury for you. You have been eating natural foods as well as your favourite food. Today you can have anything you have not eaten during the last six days. I mean anything, whatever you used to like or your desserts, or the starters, or breakfast, or lunch, dine out, or partying out. And certainly today you can have a rest from your exercise as well. And you are also not restricted from your cup of tea, meat, sugar, chocolate or other dairy products provided you have not been eating all week. You are also not restricted to any kind of drink today. If you like the things, which you did not eat during the last six days, you will feel the original taste and it will taste even better. If however you used to like the taste but today you did not enjoy it, you can give up permanently. If you think that you were restricting your amount of food, you can eat as much as you like.

How to choose the seventh day

Your seventh day can be whatever day you choose. I keep my Sunday as this is a non working day for my wife, the children and I as well. Plan the day before, what you are going to cook, who is going to cook and when are you going to eat, morning, noon or evening. Today you are celebrating the success of your new routine. Treat yourself as a star. Clean your house as if some guests are coming. Cook your dinner and display it on the table, light a candle. Have a shower, put your dinner suit on. Thank yourself for your success and enjoy your meal. If you have any party celebrations during your six days consider it as your seventh day and start again. The more you enjoy your life's events, the less you are going to eat. The time will go quicker and you will be a happier, slimmer and more active person. You will not carry the burden of dieting with you.

Habits

We all have some kind of habits, some are good and some are bad. Bad habits are easy to adapt and good habits are not, because of ignorance. It is not easy to stop a habit, whether it is good or bad. But it is very easy to slip into another. Eating is also a habit; you are only changing your habit of eating to eating healthily. You are not going on a dieting mission, so you are not doing anything temporarily. You are not doing any strenuous exercise; you are only walking, which is normal for any human beings. As I explained earlier, we have a four-chambered heart and four appendages and we have got to make-work from them.

When we do anything regularly it soon becomes a habit, and if you get into a good habit that becomes a blessing. Children adopt habits from others and definitely from their parents and carers. Leave them a fortune of good habits and they will remember you always.

Six weeks later

You will not need to weigh yourself, as you know that you are on your way to success. You are feeling happier and healthier. If you want to check your success, you can put yourself to a test. Try to do the shoe laces again, as you tried in the beginning, look at yourself in the mirror and look at your curves and speak aloud to yourself your success so far and what is remaining. Weigh yourself. At this time you are supposed to be weighing 2 kilos less than the last time. You will be feeling happier and healthier than before. You can celebrate your success. The way you are going, you will cut down 50 grams of your weight every day. The weight you are going to lose will be uniform.

Six months later

Repeat this process after six months. By this time you will be about 6-8 kilos less than the last time. This will show your and my success. You will feel happier and healthier. You will notice that you are not getting minor ailments like flu, headaches and general body aches. There will not be any sign of sadness as you have a feeling of elation in your success.

If you have diabetes or hypertension, you will need to visit your doctor to review your medicine and have some blood investigations done, as your blood lipid, blood sugar and blood urea will come down; you need lower doses of medicine or may not need it at all. Everything you have been doing will become your habit by now.

One year after

You can compare your older photographs; you will feel that instead of getting one year older you will look five years younger. You will look slimmer, healthier and happier. There will not be any circles around your eyes, any old acne marks will fade away and you face will be shiny and eyes glittery. You will not have any health problems and will have cut down all the medicine if you are having any.

You will be weighing about two stone less than last time. Usually seventy percent of over weight people are only one and a half stone heavier. Once they get to their ideal weight, a further reduction in weight will start to be a problem. At that stage it gets harder to lose more weight as our body absorbs more energy from food, which is now less than it was last year. Even then you are not going to change your habits of eating healthily, as it was not easy to learn them in the beginning.

And after

Everyday wake up in the morning and thank yourself. You are living a healthy and happy life. You are a healthy mind in a healthy body and you are always ready to face the world. Now the problems of the world became less and whatever they are, they are easy to solve, and each day becomes easy.

You do not need to weigh yourself, your mirror tells you the truth. If you weigh yourself and your weight has gone up, nothing to worry, as it will never stay the same. It will differ from day to day and morning to evening. You know how to adjust your weight, just as a ship does not move constantly in one direction, the captain has to adjust it all the time to keep to the final destination.

Why I cannot lose weight quicker

I do not want to wait for one year to be the weight I want to be. Why can't I lose weight quicker than that?

Because the quicker you lose weight, the quicker you will gain afterwards. You can lose weight quickly; there is nothing impossible in this.

If you carry on with your normal routine and do not eat anything apart from drinking water, you can lose two stone in 40 days, but you will be ill by that time. Medical recommendations for minimum calorie intake are 500 calories per day. If you consume 500 calories per day, which are a full naan bread with 100 grams of alu bhaji and a glass of orange, you can lose the same amount of weight in eighty days. The rest is up to you how you maintain your weight. If you choose this way, then I would recommend only eating fruits and vegetables and nothing else. This is the only food which can give you enough energy and all the vitamins, carbohydrates and fibre.

5 a day

Try to eat as many fruit and vegetables as you can, all the time, in all your meals. Break the routine of five a day, there is no restriction on eating more.

There is no fixed time to eat fruits. As promised earlier, be broad-minded and eat whenever you want to eat. Eat as much as you want to eat, and eat wherever you want to eat. Fruits can be eaten raw and are probably more nutritious in their raw, fresh state. Fruits and nuts obviously can be eaten raw, as well as the vegetables we eat in salads, including grated carrots and beetroot, and other vegetables not normally included in salads. Onions and garlic can be eaten raw. Grains can be flaked and eaten raw as in Muesli. Pulses may become easily digestible if you first allow them to sprout. They will sprout after being soaked and kept moist and warm for a few days. Peas and lentils sprout readily and are surprisingly sweet.

Balance your vegetable intake between the orange/red and green varieties. The more colourful your choice the healthier it usually is and, as an easy rule, the darker and brighter the colour of the vegetable the more vitamins, minerals and fibre they usually contain. For example, compare lettuce with the deep dark green of spinach or the bright orange of carrots.

The more starchy vegetables such as corn, butternut, pumpkin, peas, root vegetables and sweet potatoes should also be balanced with the less starchy vegetables such as courgettes, green beans, spinach, broccoli and cauliflower.

Friends and parties

A good friend is not the one who provides expensive junk food in abundance, but the one who provides a nutritious and enjoyable meal. A good friend is someone who tells you the truth, but in a sweeter way than telling a lie. Ignore all the comments on your weight made by your friends. It does not matter if their comments are good or bad; just go by your own instincts. Asking a friend "does my bum looks bigger?" is not going to make any difference; rather it is going to make a rift in your friendship.

Parties

A party means an occasion of happiness. Eating unnatural food and stuffing your face with the wrong calories and making yourself ill is not the idea of having a good time. If you go to such parties, enjoy your drink and meals by consuming food as slowly as can and try to taste every bit of the food, so that you know exactly what to provide when you organise your own parties.

Doctor

A General Practitioner is the doctor who is generally overseeing and supporting health and medical care in the community.

He is the most expensive and responsible worker of the community. Usually the NHS spends £150 for one consultation. You can imagine the expenditure of the patient who is under regular care of a doctor. A General Practitioner's duty includes providing you with the services, which can prevent you falling ill. It is better if you visit the doctor when you are not ill and get his advice on preventing ill health, rather than go to doctor when you are ill.

His difficulty is that he is applying only what he has learnt in those years studying books. He is applying the data taken from people like you. He does not know what is required by you and what weight you are supposed to be. He is only going by the charts supplied to him. You are the best person to decide the weight and the size you want to be, and trust me you can if you want to.

Doctors and other health workers are human beings too. They have the same incidence and prevalence of illnesses as the rest of the population. They suffer from diabetes, hypertension and other illnesses no less than other people.

Dietician

A dietician is the healthcare professional responsible for the planning and managing of a patient's diet in a hospital and providing dietary advice.

He is the right person to help you and advise you about your diet, but only when you are ill, especially in diabetes.

When you are not ill there is no need for a dietician; your natural instinct is the guide to what to eat and when to eat.

Pysiotherapist

A physiotherapist is a health care professional who assesses the physical function of the body and helps to restore and maintain as normal a function as possible.

He is a great help after sporting injuries, accidental injuries, certain operations and some long-term illnesses.

In normal circumstances you are the best person to look after yourself. Only you can look after yourself, no one else can. It is all right to take advice from someone when you need to.

Celebrities

Our celebrities are those who are paid loads of money for their work.

They become role models for us for their work, for their image and we are always ready to listen to them. The advertising companies advertise their product and make them richer. I am afraid in this process the general population are never considered for their health or wealth. For example, one of my favourite players and a great footballer advertises a brand of crisps. I can never imagine a footballer eating crisps, especially if he is to maintain the highest level of fitness. Other examples are advertisement of detox regimes, videos and drinks.

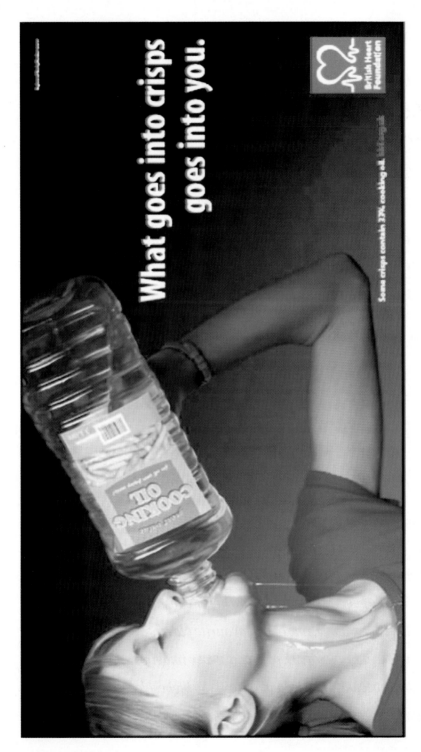

British Heart Foundation has kindly permitted to include this poster into this book

Advertisement

This recent poster by the British Heart Foundation is showing awareness that no fat be it liquid form or solid is good for you. This is the first time I have seen such kind of an advertisement, which can actually help in solving diet issues. If more of these kind of posters were distributed all over the world it is going to be a big help to reduce the morbidity and mortality due to health illnesses; where butter (ghee) was the cause of heart illnesses now oil is being misinterpreted as healthier than butter.

Ageing

Ageing is a continuous slow process. We count it in years, months and weeks. Every day we change but the process is so slow that we do not notice every day. We only notice it when we look at old pictures.
There is a difference between being old in years, looking old and feeling old. The latter is worse.

The factors, which make the difference, are obesity, illness and worries. As we get older hiding those ageing features, like wrinkles, is not going to make us any younger, but certainly being and feeling healthy and feeling younger makes you younger than your counterparts of the same age. Our idea is not to add years to your life, but to put life into those years, which you have.

Beauty

Beauty is the combination of features according to your liking. Many things are accounted by how you look, feel and think. Most of the times, it is superficial interaction and a quick judgement.

Every one of us is made the same way and every one has the same features as others. It is the same as age, there is a difference in being beautiful, looking beautiful and feeling beautiful. Healthy eyes and lips make people look more attractive, but sunken eyes and sunken cheeks are due to starvation, which definitely do not make you beautiful.
Beauty products can make you look beautiful, but only temporarily. But if you are healthy and cheerful it means you have done much to improve your looks. Beauty products are not going to make much difference, but definitely being in good shape makes you more attractive.

Most foods reflect on your body. Meat and meat products make you look like bacon. And if you eat milk and milk products you look imbalanced and muscular. If you eat cakes and biscuits you will be soft and gooey. If you eat vegetables and fruits you will look fresh and shiny at all times.

Skin

Skin reflects the state of your health. Your skin identifies many diseases. Facial skin is the main worry for young people. Pimples and acne appear at the start of puberty, due to hormonal changes. If the health is good and the diet is free of any additions of salt, sugar and fat, only a few spots will appear but even then they will not leave any residual marks. Everything required for a healthy skin is obtained from your diet of fruit and vegetables, there is nothing else your skin requires other than fresh air and exercise. Skin absorbs many chemicals. They are absorbed by the skin and circulate and are distributed in the body, giving man some side effects. Many beauty products are well known to cause cancers.

Skin can be stretched but cannot be returned back to its former state because it looses its elasticity. That's why stretch marks don't go away. It is better if you stay at your original weight than to put on and reduce it down by dieting. After giving birth, stretch marks appear called Stria. They are due to hormonal changes, but regular exercise before, during and after pregnancy make them less and less visible.

Me

After I had been to my father's funeral I lost sleep, my concentration and lost interest in everything. Literally I was in depression. I will share my thoughts with you, which I have never even shared with my wife. Being a doctor I could not understand what happened to my father.

Why him? Will I die the same way, and will my son go through the same pain, which I went through?

All these questions were going through my brain. Even as a doctor I did not have any answers. One day an idea came to my mind. Worrying about being dead was not going to help anyone. I decided I was going to use my skills to help the people I love and started to put myself into research.

My research

I did not know where to start. Every research needs money and I did not have any. And already there is plenty of research that has been going on for many years. The government, the charitable organisations and the pharmaceutical companies usually sponsor any research. My criteria did not fit into any one of them. So I did not have any hope. Even if I got the support, it is not going to help anyone other than the sponsor. There is only one criterion when carrying out research, and that is to earn money. For example if a cereal producing company is going to sponsor you for research, either you have to prove that their cereal is healthy for you or you have to produce a new product, which you can prove is healthy. You will not dare to speak against your sponsor.

I set on my own and easy way and found the easy solution. I compiled a PowerPoint presentation and presented it to my family. Everyone liked the way of leading a different life. I presented a few seminars, which became popular in India.

Coming back to England, life became busy again; I was studying as well as working. I did not get any time to do any more seminars and I could not promote them, as this was not a business enterprise.

My wife gave me the idea to put everything into a book. Not to make a profit, but to raise awareness. It is now in your hands.

What went wrong with my father's health?

If I find the answer to that question, then it would be the solution for others. He was intelligent, physically and mentally strong. I am the oldest son in the family and the first to graduate as a doctor in the area where I lived, so I should have some idea what went wrong. He belonged to a family which was not well off, and his idea was to come out of that situation, which he did successfully. He educated himself, got a job and moved out of the village. There were three main needs for a family to live: on roti (bread), (kapda) clothes to wear and (makaan) a house to live in, and he kept the roti as a priority.

He provided us with every kind of food which was available and which was thought healthy. He knew milk was healthy; apart from buying milk he bought a buffalo. He only had to know that something was healthy and he would go and buy it in abundance. Mind you, I have never known him to buy any kind of junk food. Anyway in those areas where we lived junk food was not available. All the food in our house was healthy - meat, milk and eggs - and no one would have wished for more than that.

He was not a smoker and but a moderate drinker. Throughout my life I have never seen him ill, even with minor ailments. So what went wrong? That was easy to work out, it was food in abundance. Was he to blame for his own eating habits? Definitely not. It was the people around him telling him what was good to eat. And that's what I want to say in this book. The advertising companies tell us how the food looks, the quality of the food and the taste of the food we have, and even if you try everything as a sample it can provide you with enough calories to live on. Food in abundance is the true factor. You will not see an obese man in prisoner of war camps, in draughts and flood regions.

Addiction

The rule of addiction is that you can be addicted to anything only when you have it. You cannot be addicted to anything, which is not available to you. When you have a first cup of tea, you need the second. When you have the first cigarette, you needed the second one, and that's how you become addicted to smoking. It's the same for food and alcohol. The best way to get rid of addiction is stop taking it completely, because you do not need those things, which you are addicted to. Do not buy them at all. Stop any addiction you have you do not wish to pass it on to your children. Change all the habits for today, tomorrow and forever and pass your good habits on to the generations to come.

Obesity and children

Children with a weight problem are all too aware that society doesn't view them favourably. As they get fat, they become more reclusive and go out less and do less exercise.

Young children who are obese are vulnerable to being bullied at school. At the same time, many children who are bullied, instead of telling their problems to parents or a teacher, turn to comfort eating because of their unhappiness. This adds to their problems.

Diets high in processed foods are causing bad behaviour and learning difficulties in children.

With a young child you have the advantage of a blank sheet and you can educate that child's palate, habits and mindset. Even as they grow older and more independent, by establishing a taste for real food early on you have done valuable 'programming' which can be relied upon to create a healthy framework, even if they stray from time to time.

If you have only recently overhauled the family's eating habits, however, and older children are being re-educated, you may have more of a struggle on your hands. The trick is not to give up and to be consistent in your approach. If you keep going, eventually you will make a difference. You will just need to go slowly and keep praising any positive changes that are made.

Imagination

Six months ago I imagined this book I also imagined what it would look like, how big it is going to be and what it is going to be about. Today it is in your hands, and I can tell you that it is exactly as I imagined. I wish for you to do the same. Imagine what you will look like in six months time, how healthy, slim, active and full of life you are going to be. And I am sure you are going to achieve that.

This my revolutionary idea

According to the RSPCA, 750 million farm animals are reared in the UK each year. The huge demand for meat, eggs and dairy products has encouraged farmers to use intensive methods of farming. Usually this means animals are kept in a limited space with little opportunity to roam outside and look for their own food.

If these animals were not farmed there would not be any beef, milk, eggs and dairy products. As a result, I would predict an 80% reduction in mortality and morbidity from heart diseases.

Then why do we not encourage this? Because of one simple reason, marketing and economy. There is a high demand for these products. If there were a comparable demand for fruit and vegetables farmers would have to grow plants. More vegetation means more rain and more rain means more life.

Suggestions

Use all farming land to grow fruit plants and vegetable plants. Instead of using land for animal feed you can grow a wide variety of fruits. You can grow fruits even in your home garden.

If you are a teacher, teach about plants, if you are a banker give more loans and subsidies to farmers to grow more plants and vegetables. If you are a businessman, the fruit business, is growing, you already know that. If you go in to the food stores, fruit and vegetables are dearer. A law of economics is that availability is indirectly proportional to the price. If fruits and vegetables are more available these would be sold cheaper.

Eating basic food without any luxurious cooking can save us from getting ill and avoid going to hospital and save the NHS money.

Fasting once a week can save us from getting fat and ultimately saves food for others. "Back to Basics" by Honourable Mr. John Major and Mahatma Gandhi's slogan "Simple Living and High Thinking" are true to its words.

The big stores are producing their own brands of processed foods, which are high in salt, fat and sugar contents. These are cheap and the stores are claiming that you can shop cheaper in their stores compared to others. It is better to buy a healthy product in small quantities than to buy cheaper food in bulk, which is unhealthy.

Your Promise

Name   :

Age   :

Sex   :

Address   :

Height   :

Weight   :

Blood pressure :

How you feel   :

I promise to stay healthy all my life

Comments

My Idols

John Major

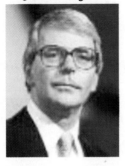

"It is time to get back to basics: to self-discipline and respect for the law, to consideration for others, to accepting responsibility for yourself and your family, and not shuffling it off on the state" - 1993

Mahatma Gandhi

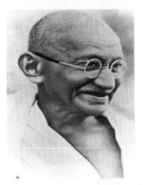

"Mahatma Gandhi spent his entire life denouncing and campaigning against non-vegetarian food and alcohol. Gandhi taught respect for animals as well as humans, a non-exploitative relationship to the environment, the elimination of poverty, the limitation of personal wealth and possessions, and non-violence applied at all levels from the interpersonal to relationships between states."

"Our children are not eating enough fruit"

Mr Tony Blair
Prime Minister of the UK

To the honourable prime minister

Ref: "Our children are not eating enough fruit & child obesity"
I appreciate your concern about children not eating enough fruit. In my opinion, it is the obesity problem that needs closer attention. Current UK statistics reveal that more than 30% of children are either overweight or obese. The prime reason being unhealthy eating habits and inadequate consumption of fruit is only one of these habits.

Does anyone have an effective proven solution for child obesity? I am afraid that just by outlining the agenda on national media with statements like "Children are not eating enough fruit" is not helping to find any solution.

All this ambiguity and worry has inspired me to invent my own theory to this problem in the form of my first book "Healthy Hearts".

Everyone should have the freedom to eat any food of their choice, but only once and after they have eaten five or more fruits in that day. Similarly, before they consume any other form of liquid, they need to make sure they have finished drinking two litres of water in that day.

I strongly believe that if this proposal is declared through the media, at least 50% of this obesity problem to be rectified. Further reformation of school meals is the classic answer to this issue. Only supply fruits, vegetables and water in schools leaving children to eat cooked meals at home. Compared to the cost of cooking food, fruit is going to be much cheaper and healthier and easier to transport from farm to the mouth. This is my proposal to you and I would like you to consider this option and also have in mind as to the place in which this society is heading. As you are still in power you will not only be remembered as the prime minister who succeeded talks and came to a peace reform with the IRA, but someone as a person who is doing something about the future of our children and our country. As a father who also has children like myself. I am asking for your interaction with this current situation.

This book has objectives, it has been written with an aim so why cannot it be part of our children's curriculum? Why should there be TV programmes, statistics or children being used as guinea pigs? Why cannot this be drummed into us and passed on from generation to generation?
I sincerely thank you for your time in reading this letter and I eagerly await your reply and proposals.

Dr.Surinder Singh

Useful website addresses;

www.bhf.org.uk

www.netdoctor.co.uk

www.nhsdirect.nhs.uk

www.bbc.co.uk

www.dfes.gov.uk

www.diabetes.org.uk

www.dh.gov.uk

www.dardni.gov.uk

www.nottingham.ac.uk

www.kidshealth.org

www.aatl.co.uk

10 DOWNING STREET
LONDON SW1A 2AA

From the Direct Communications Unit

17 October 2006

Dr. Surinder Singh

Dear Dr. Singh

The Prime Minister has asked me to thank you for your recent letter, the contents of which will be carefully noted.

Mr. Blair has asked that your letter be passed to the Department of Health which has particular responsibility for the matter you raise so that they are also aware of your views.

Yours sincerely

R. SMITH